The Longevity Book first published by Brock Creative Media in 2019. Photography by Kale Brock, Mitch Imgraben & Edmund Renew.

Design by Kristen Cowell.

Brock Creative Media Sydney, NSW, Australia

brockcreativemedia.com

The Longevity Book

Kale Brock is an award nominated writer, speaker & filmmaker. With a passion for creative storytelling and for health and wellness, his works, such as The Gut Movie, The Gut Healing Protocol & The Longevity Film have inspired many to change their lives for the better by challenging commonplace health advice.

Learn more at kalebrock.com

Dedicated to the open, curious minds of the world

"Moral certainty is always a sign of cultural inferiority. The more uncivilized the man, the surer he is that he knows precisely what is right and what is wrong.The truly civilized man is always skeptical and tolerant, in this field as in all others. His culture is based on "I am not too sure."

- H.L. Mencken

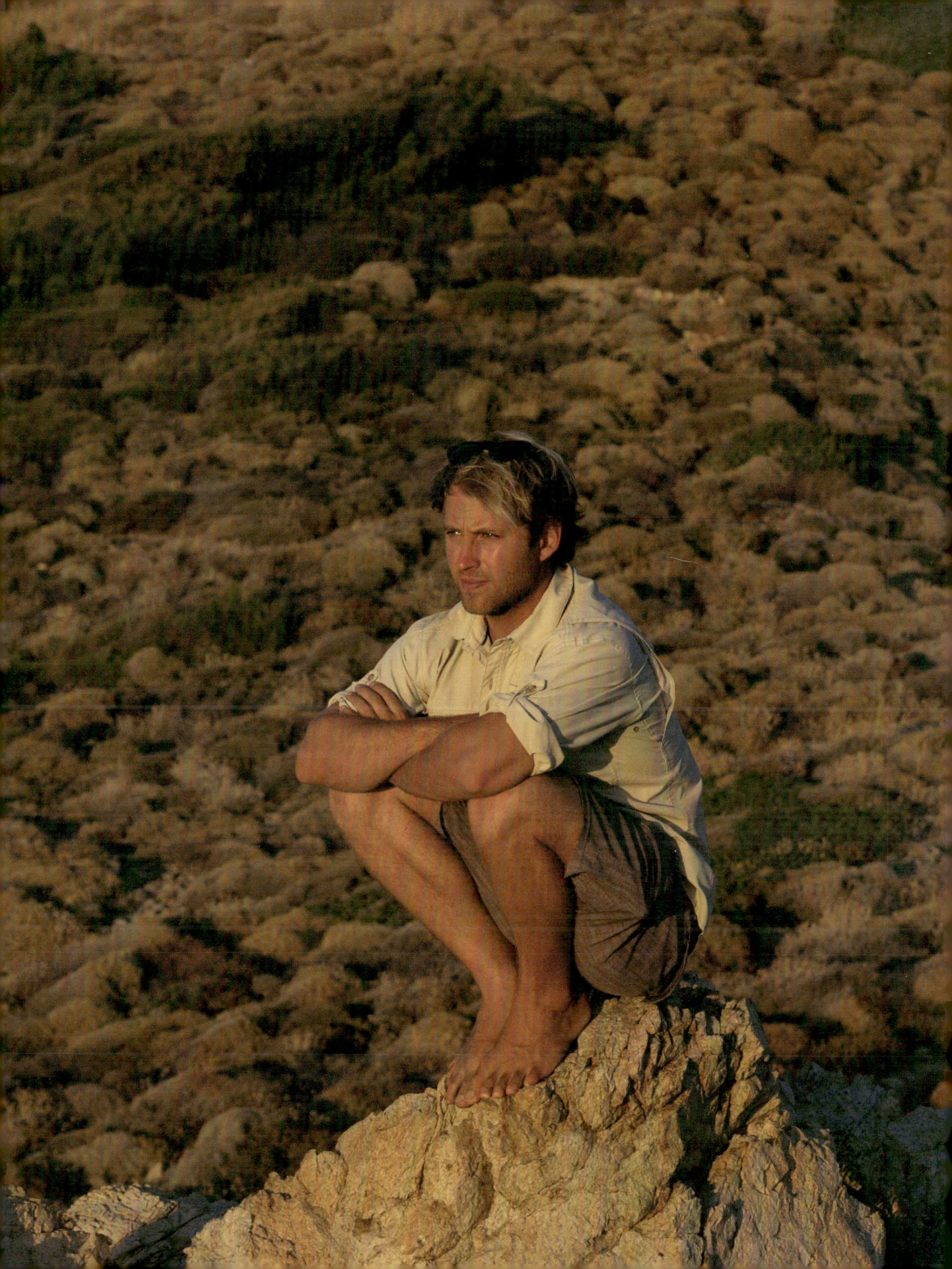

Munich airspace, Lufthansa Flight 1753

The late European sun shines a golden light over the green pastures of Munich, Germany. I gaze out the window of the plane contentedly at the cultivated agricultural fields interspersed with classical European architecture made even more romantic from above. I'm in a deeply introspective mood. A warm positive light, perhaps soaked up from the sun's favourable aesthetic at this time of the afternoon, fills my thoughts as I reflect on the last month's journey across the globe.

I've been following an intense production schedule for my new documentary, The Longevity Film. In my second movie investigating health and wellness I've been visiting the world's longest lived, healthiest, and I would now say happiest, cultures and beyond capturing the story on camera, this experience has totally shattered my perspective on life, work and of course, health.

The very moral structures upon which I have designed my life have been thrust into a metaphorical and literal spotlight (in the film) as I was challenged, constantly, with the observation of a way of life that is almost the complete opposite of what I've been doing for the past 9 years since I finished school. I'm the health guy, the microbiome writer, the speaker on all things gut and yet my 'science' of getting healthy only scratches the surface of what I've learned whilst living with the people of Okinawa (Japan), Loma Linda (California) and Ikaria (Greece).

Longevity cultures were identified in the early 2000s by a team of researchers at National Geographic. I spoke with one of the researchers in California, Nick Buettner, who shared the initial process that sparked what would become the 'blue zone' project.

"Researchers in Sardinia were recording the incidence of centenarians. Every time they found one they would put a blue dot on a map and eventually they found this region that had a lot of blue dots. They put a big blue circle around it so we just called it 'the blue zone'. We found five blue zones around the world; Sardinia, Italy, Okinawa, Japan, Ikaria, Greece, Loma Linda in California and the Nicoya Peninsula in Costa Rica. They have low rates of middle aged mortality, they're reaching 100 at rates ten times higher than we're doing it here in the 'West' and I think more importantly they do it with a fraction of the disease. "

Statistically, people in these cultures spend far less time in hospital, take much less medication and are notably more likely to reach their 90s and the golden age of 100 than everybody else.

The next question of course was, *how were they doing it?*

The researchers went on to identify key elements[1] of the people's lifestyle in these regions which they believed were contributing to their incredible wellbeing.

I observed common practices in person whilst visiting Okinawa, Loma Linda and Ikaria, and I will share my perspectives with you in this book. I have named them *The Four Pillars Of Longevity & Wellness.*

They are:

Nutrition
Community
Movement
& Attitude.

And together they make up the concept of balance. Balance is key here, because each of these pillars needs to be appreciated in order to attain excellent wellbeing and longevity.

1. See https://www.bluezones.com/2016/11/power-9/

You can have the perfect diet, if you try hard enough. You can eat a seasonal, organic and local diet tailored perfectly to your genetic needs at different stages of your life, however if you only appreciate this one pillar of longevity and wellness, whilst ignoring the others, the foundations of your being will be shaky.

If we are to ride the wave of life successfully, without getting sick and to a ripe old age of 90+, then we need some really good foundations in place. I like to use the analogy of surfing a wave (as you do!). There are numerous components that must come together in order to ride a wave successfully such as leg strength, core strength, mobility and coordination. If one of these components is misfiring or inadequate, the entire ride is compromised. However, if they are all performing optimally, they achieve excellent *balance*.

Balance is what we need to get well *and stay well* for the rest of our life. This is not just about living a long time. Although that can be achieved, what we do want to ensure is that we have great *quality* in our years. Unfortunately right now, we do not have that.

"*For the first time in history, our children are expected to live a sicker life and to die younger than their parents.*

-Dr Mark Hyman

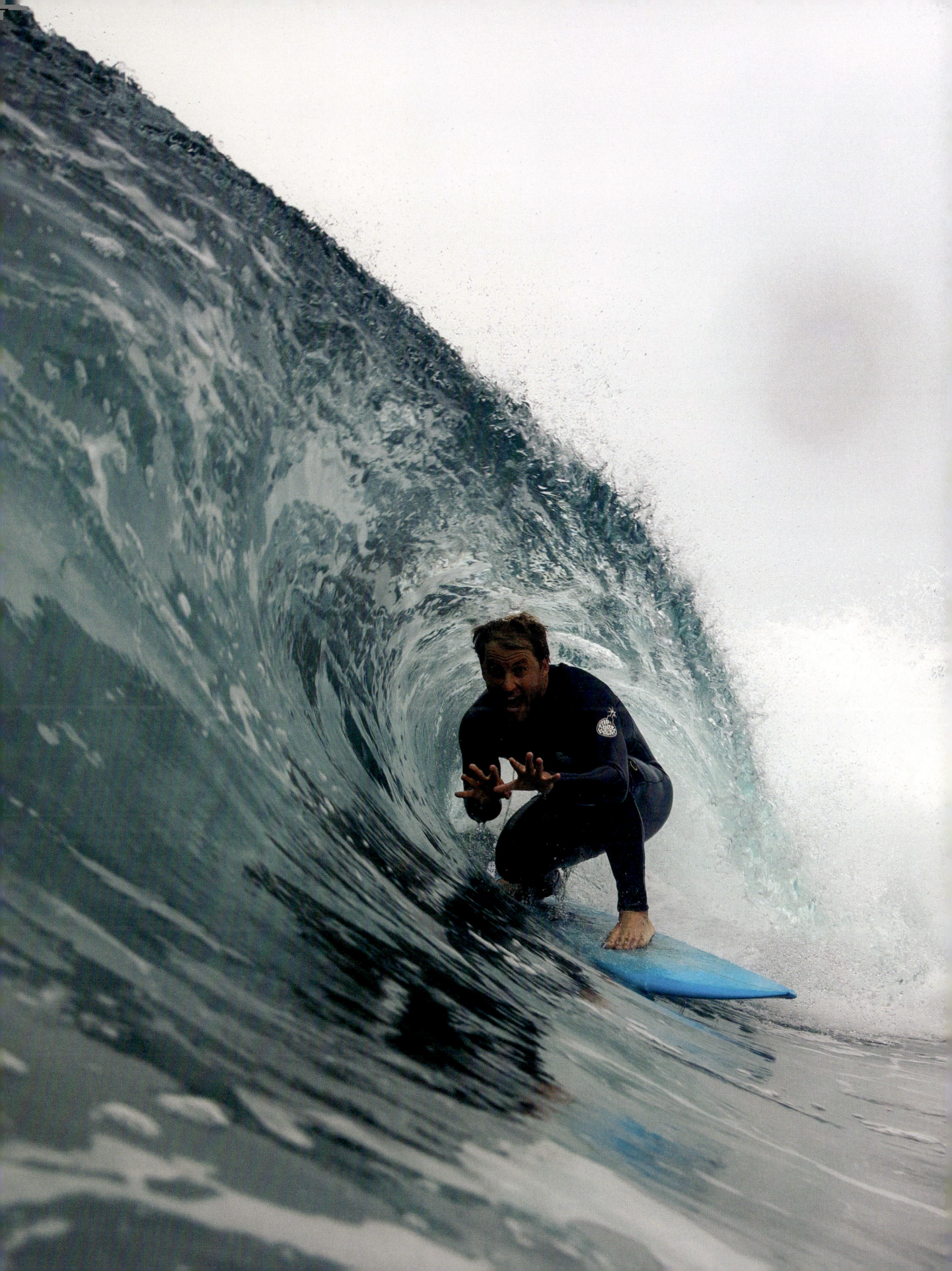

This is where modern medicine is failing us at this time. We know a lot about keeping unhealthy people alive for a long time, but we know very little about getting them *well* again so that they can live with independence and integrity.

Throughout my time with the longevity cultures, I met with 100 year olds who still lived independently, who dressed themselves, cooked for themselves, danced, drank tea with friends and walked staircases daily! And they were sharp intellectually. As one of the original blue zone researchers, Nick Buettner, put it, "you tend to see a lot more cerebral readiness in these cultures."

Out of all the interviews which I conducted whilst in these cultures, only one of the elderly people I met was on ongoing medication.
And it was only *one drug.*

Most of the graceful agers I spoke to weren't on any medication at all. They might have taken some for an acute condition throughout their lives, be it pneumonia or a persistent infection, but never ongoing; only for a short amount of time.

In Australia, 90% of us take some form of medication each year, 40% of us take two medications every week and 10% of us take medication *daily.* In fact, older people in the West are generally *expected* to be on multiple medications at any given time and these often come with a slew of side effects and direct negative health consequences. With these side effects often comes the need to take more medication, attend doctors visits more frequently and a decreased quality of life can be expected, which is in complete contradiction to the intention behind the medication in the first place.

"There is no disease in existence today that is the result of a deficiency of a drug."

-Dr Damian Kristof

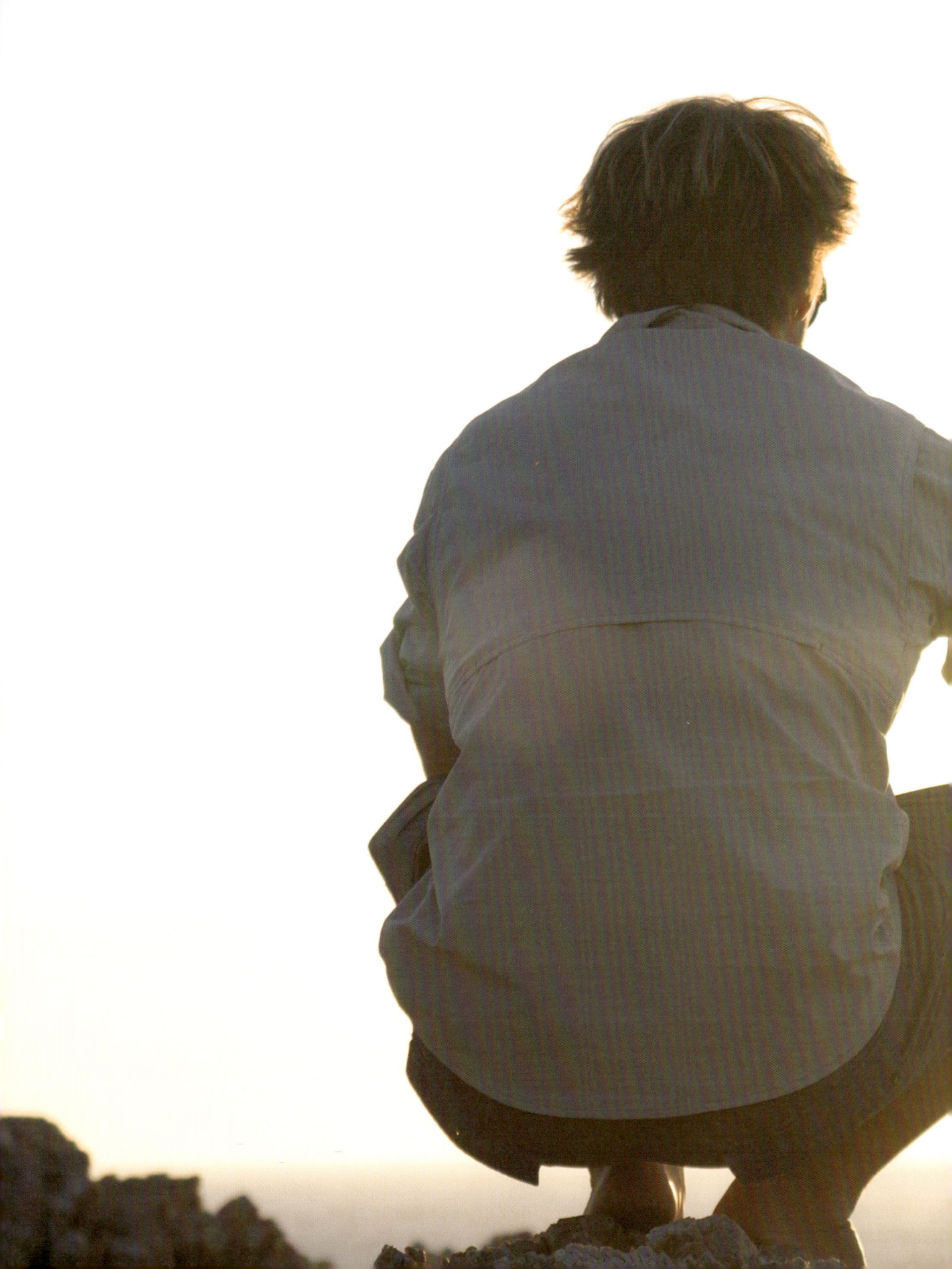

The common misconception that pharmaceuticals are required to help us live a long time is deeply embedded within most cultures outside of the blue zones. Short term pharmaceutical use can indeed be life saving, such as in the case of antibiotics when used for severe infections, however, long-term use of medications is very rarely associated with an increased quality of life. If we take into account the observations of the longevity cultures, then it may in fact be the opposite.

It may indeed be possible to add five to ten *quality years* to your life by honouring your body's needs like the people of Okinawa, Loma Linda, Ikaria, Sardinia & The Nicoya Peninsula.. And the best part about this is that *it's not hard.* It turns out that we've been led slightly astray in Western society. Our priorities are a little mixed up, that's all. We can change things around.

The people I met in the following communities were vital, energetic, happy, engaged and independent throughout their entire life. Let's meet them now.

The Longevity Cultures

Okinawa

Okinawa, Japan was my first filming location for *The Longevity Film*. It is home to the largest number of centenarians out of anywhere in the world. Although a culture clash has been ensuing since WWII with the arrival and establishment of an American army base, the people have, largely, been able to maintain their traditional lifestyles albeit with a modern twist.

Okinawans have an average life expectancy of 87 years for the women and 81 for the men. The key here is that they can expect to live 97% of their lives *free from disease*. In Australia, nearly half of all *children* are living with a chronic health condition.

Okinawans can expect to have 80% less heart disease, 75% less breast & prostate cancer and 65% less dementia.

Needless to say, this Hawaiian-esque island 2000km South-West of Tokyo is a longevity and wellness superhub.

Whilst there, I had a production schedule to match the best of them yet I may as well have left it at home. Carrying a tight schedule in these communities is like trying to trudge your way through quicksand with a heavy backpack, it only serves as a source of frustration and irritation and as your struggles intensify your situation worsens, the level of your capitulation into the mud a reflection of the level at which you refuse to let your time-related expectations fall to the wayside.

The deeply rooted patience and presence which the Okinawans brought to the community meetings and events I attended was beautiful to see.

I watched one such person, Yoshiko, who is 93 years old, navigate an incredibly active and busy day (even by middle aged standards) of karaoke, meetings, hosting me for tea and snacks, hosting her own radio show and gardening with such poise, grace and calmness I almost couldn't believe it.

Yoshiko flowed effortlessly between engaging with us on camera, preparing food, and singing and dancing on stage in front of hundreds of people from her community. There was a marked lack of urgency about her, but an equally notable sense of efficiency, flow and presence in her operation. I asked her what the secret is, I'd never seen someone of that age be so busy and nimble through such a schedule and she laughed between delicate sips of green tea whilst she delivered her thoughts.

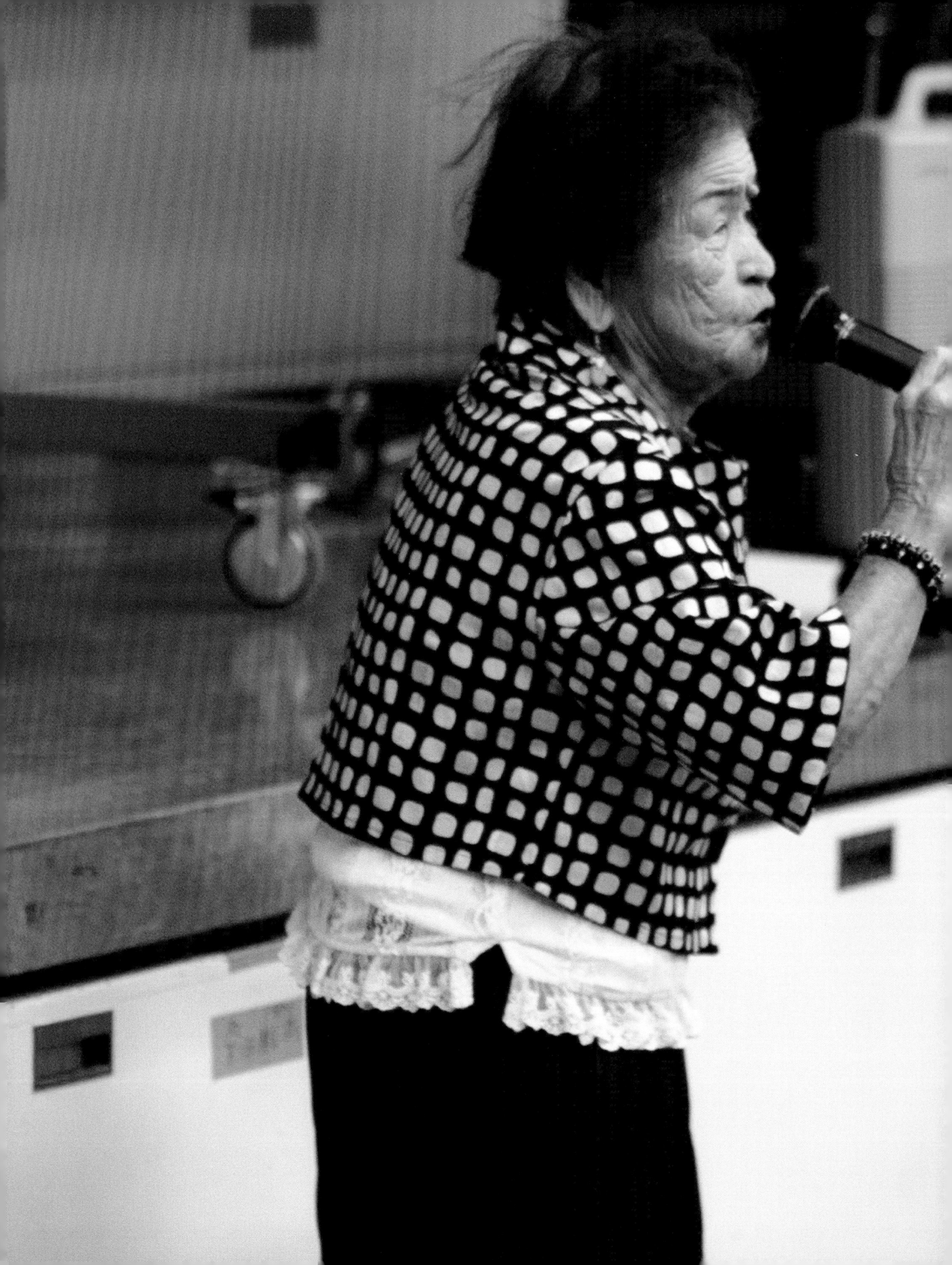

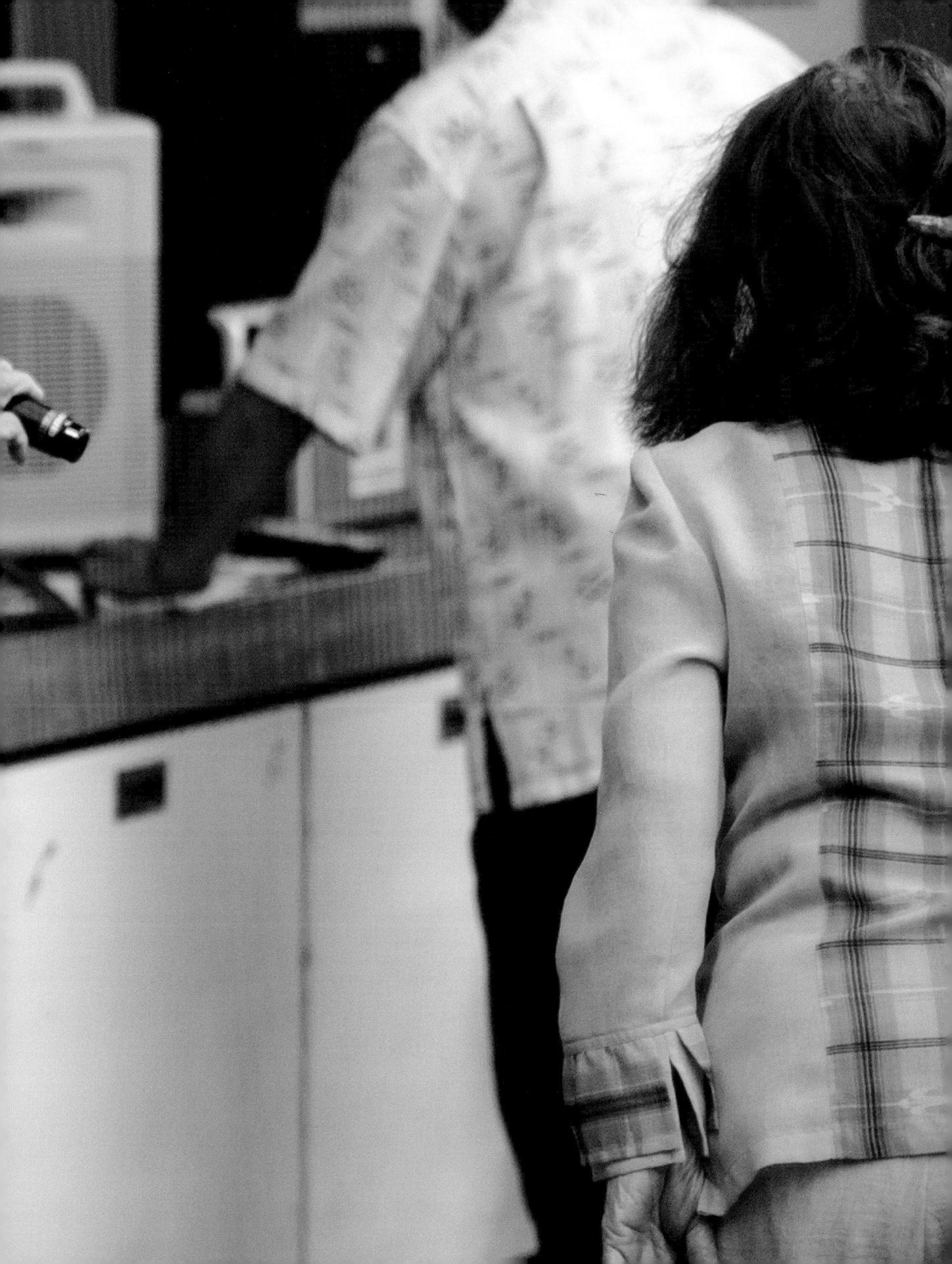

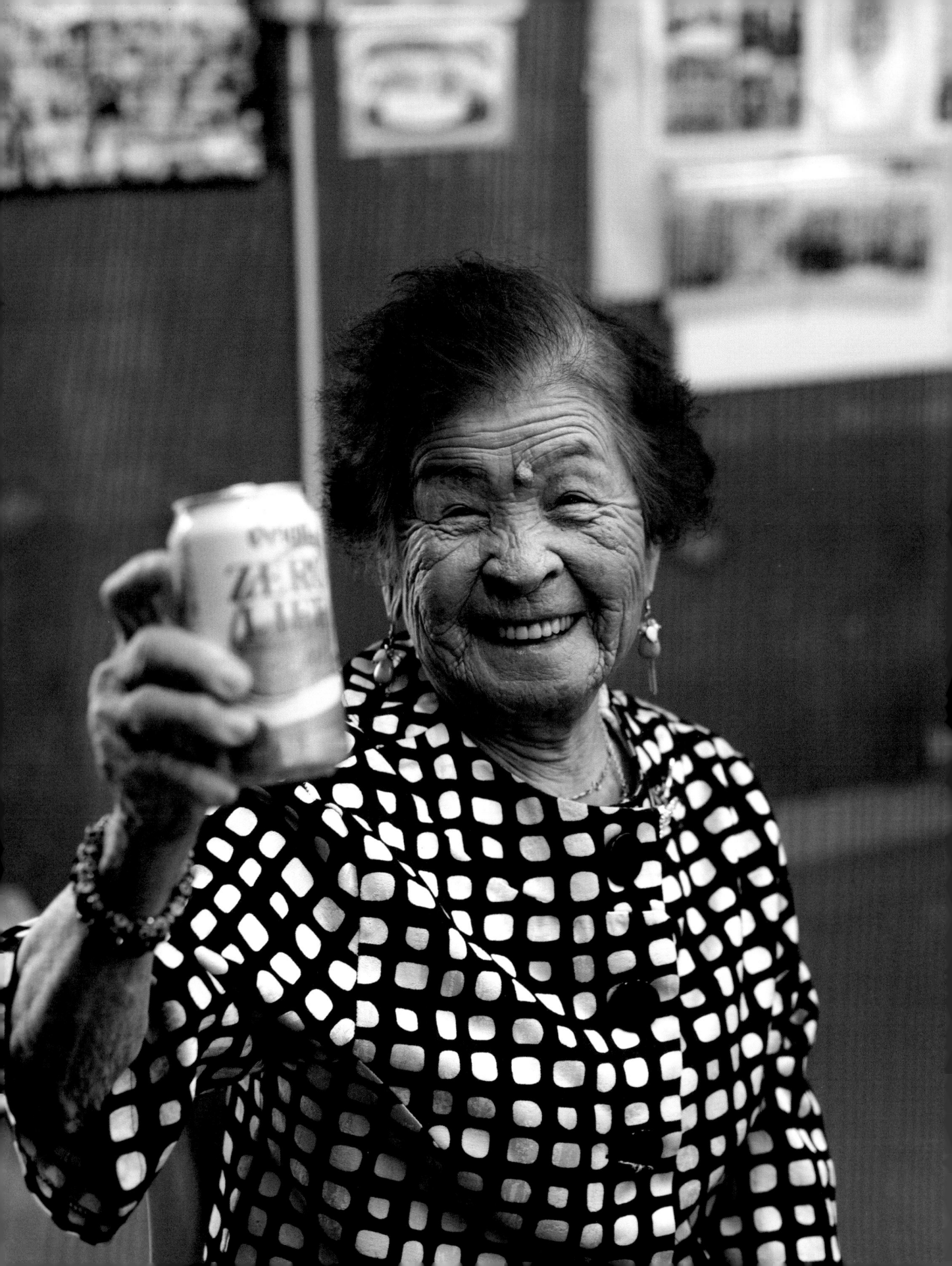

"The secret is not to think too much. I'm too busy to grow old – I don't have time for that. The doctor says I should slow down, but I don't."

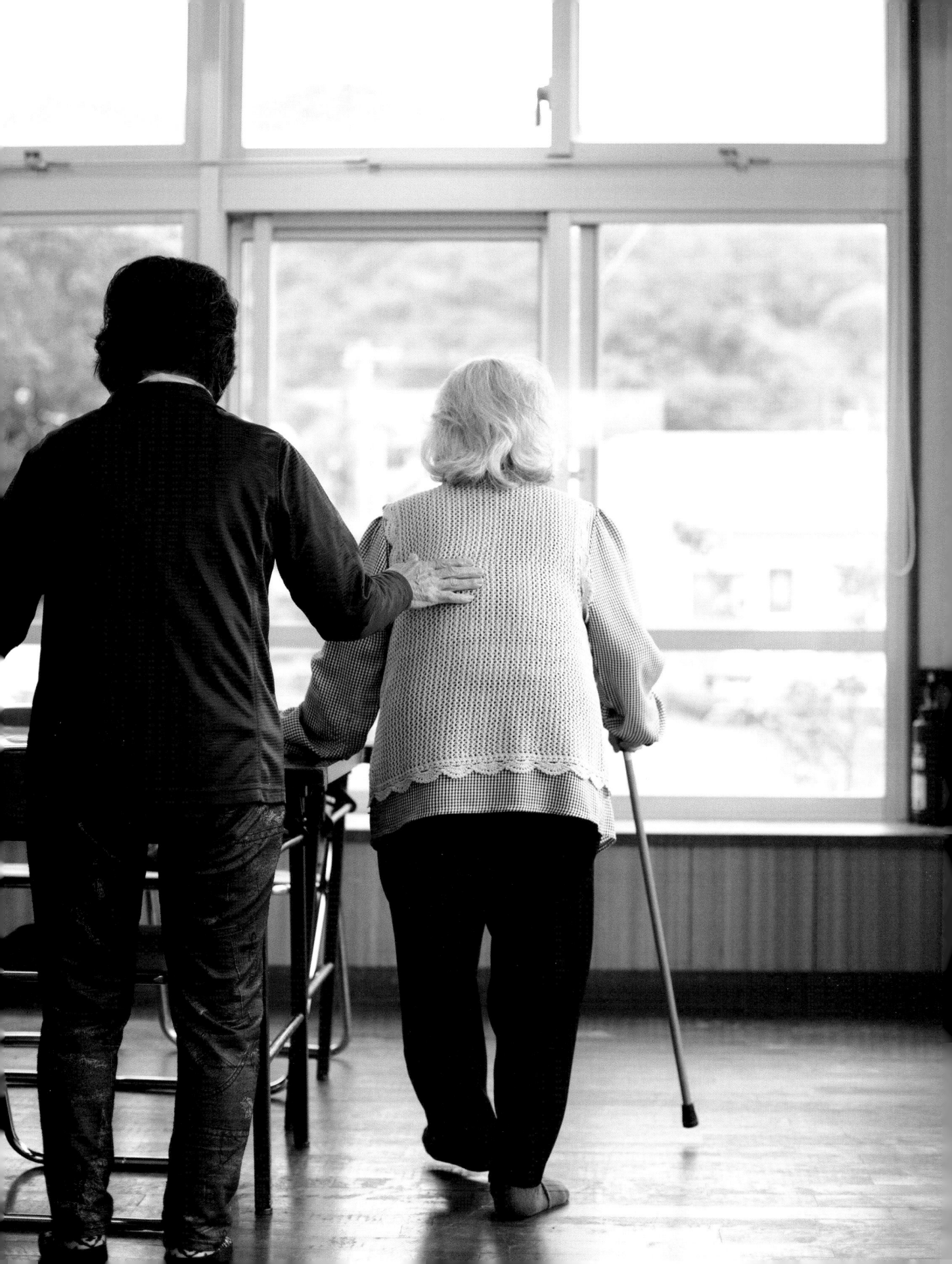

"I eat anything that I like. Mostly I enjoy vegetables. I didn't eat beef until I was 63, now I love it. But I never eat until I'm full. I only drink green tea. Nothing else, except for once a week when I am at karaoke. I have one beer on those nights."

"Do you take any medicine at all?" I inquired, curious.

"Normally I don't take any medicines. I just sleep to help feel better. Sometimes I take medicines for a cold, but mostly just sleep."

"How important are your friends?"

"I enjoy being with friends. We only talk about good things. We don't want to talk about any bad things because we want to have a good time together. I want people to feel like they have a happy experience when they meet me.

"I am very busy. Monday I go to dancing & lunch with friends. Tuesday I host my radio program. Wednesday is my singing practice. Thursday is my karaoke party. Friday always something happens. Saturday I am working in the garden all day. It's Thursday today. Let's go to karaoke."

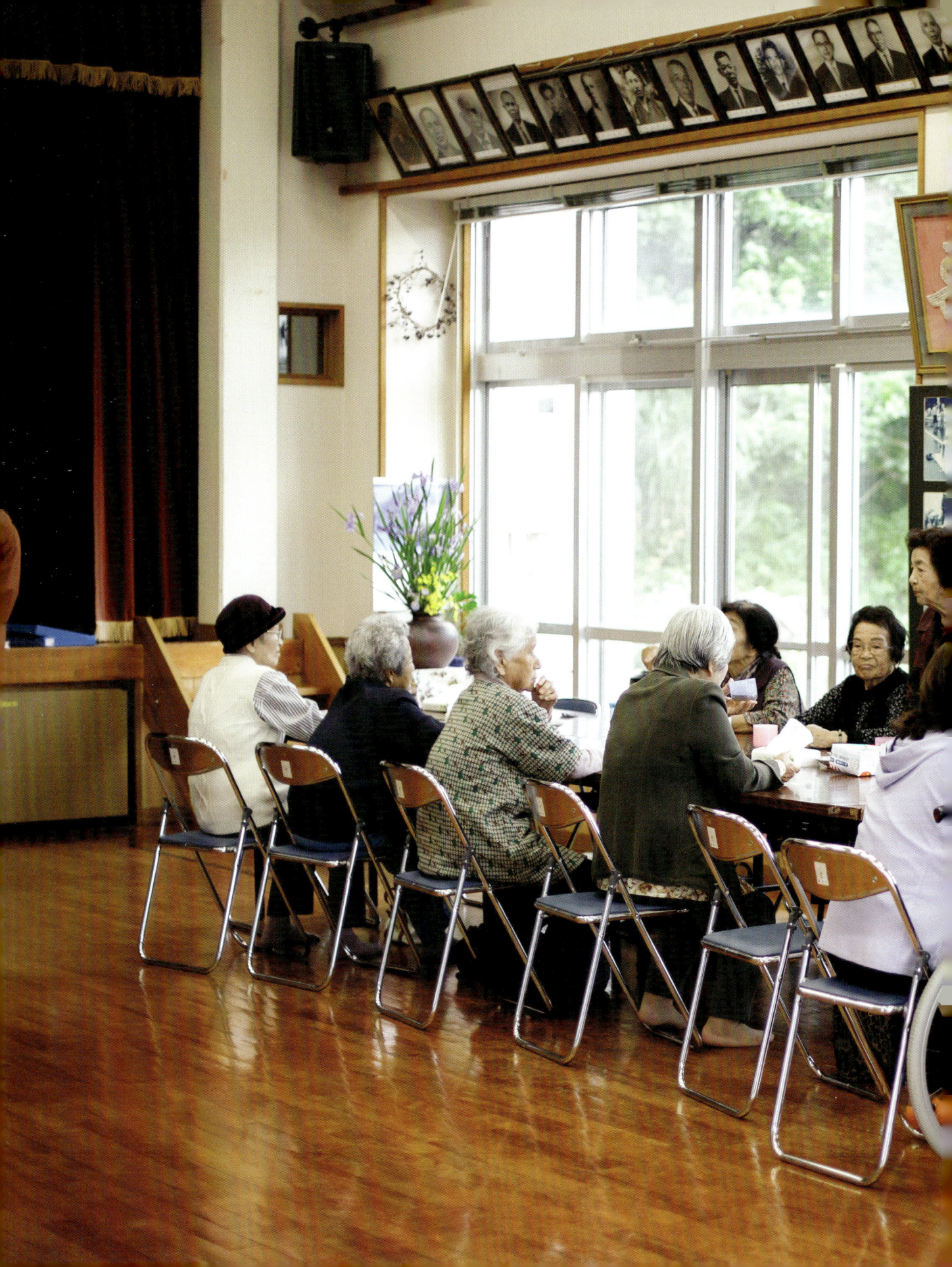

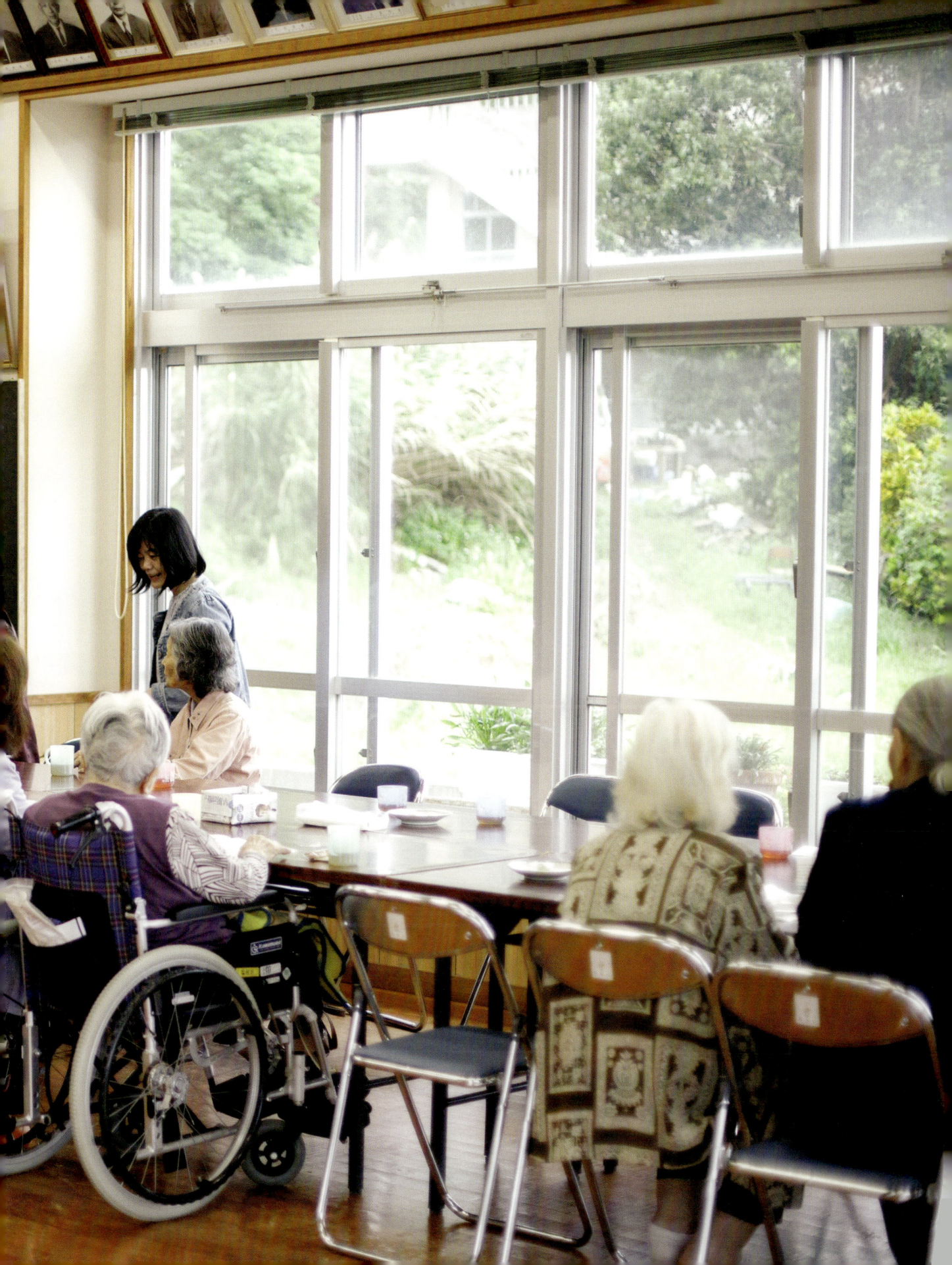

Yoshiko's schedule is insanely busy for one her age, but it's the total relaxation, the lack of urgency with which she follows it, that empowers Yoshiko to thrive.

We arrived, excited, at the unassuming karaoke club, fitted with colourful frills, disco lights and plastic-diamond speckled microphones. It quickly filled up with 5 energetic women over 90 all sipping at incongruously large mugs of beer. They raised their glasses toward us.

"Kari! *Cheers!*"

After some blunt chit chat, somewhat immune to the omnipresence of our production equipment, the ladies finally took to the stage to deliver a glorious quintet with Yoshiko, the leading woman, beaming under the lights as she embraced her solos like Gaga in *A Star Is Born.*

She was in her element, glowing even, as her and her friends delivered lines from the rolling teleprompter. When they finished she bounded off the stage with timeless grace, glanced over and said, "this is the reason for growing old."

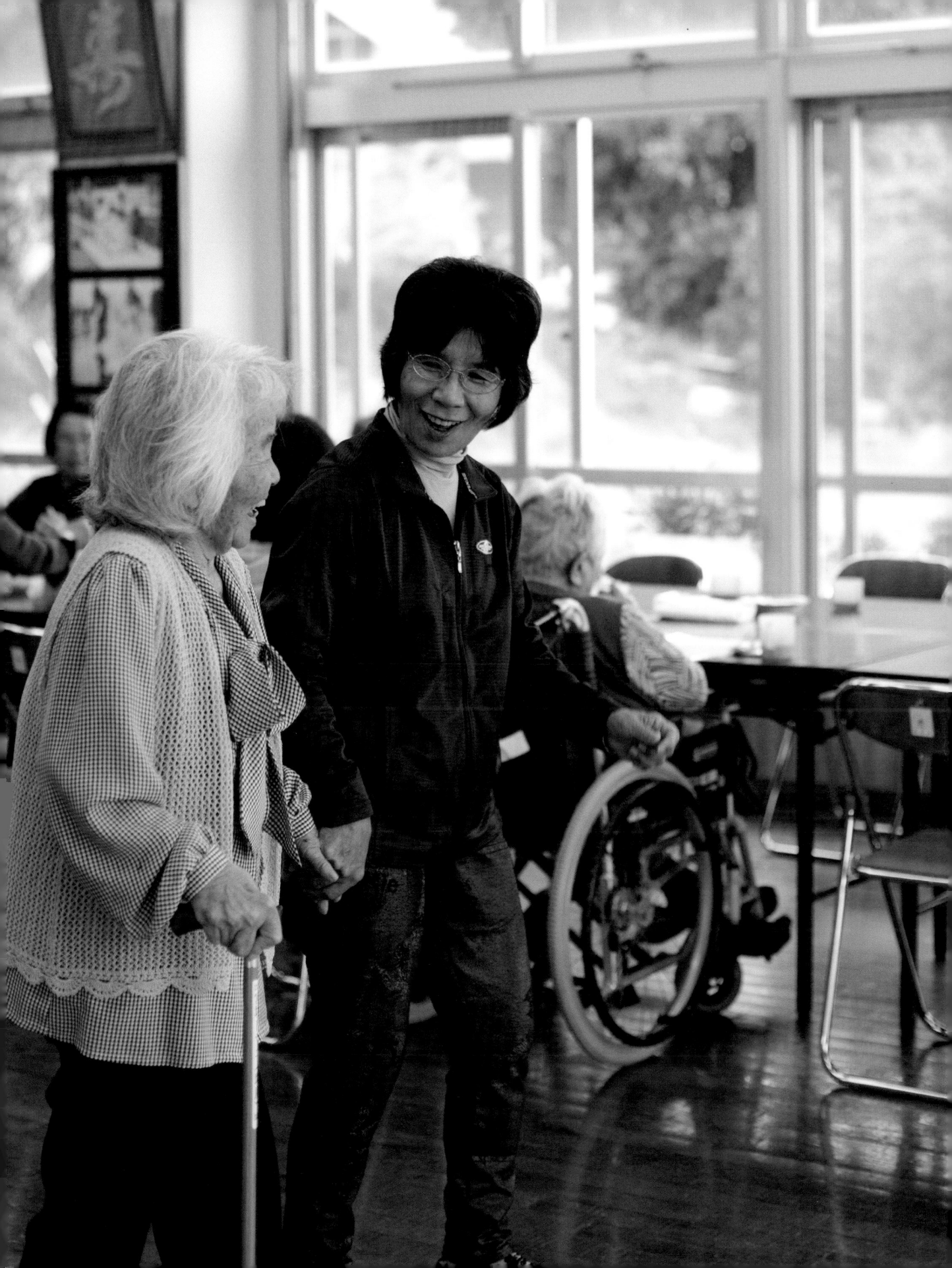

Loma Linda, California

Arguably the most interesting longevity hotspot in the world is Loma Linda, California. Every single person I shared my itinerary with baulked at the USA component, presuming that we were filming the 'fat, sick and nearly dead' whilst there. However, I came across in Loma Linda one of the most curious anomalies I've ever had the pleasure of considering. Loma Lindan people have an average life expectancy that is *ten years longer* than their American counterparts and yet, geographically, and socially to an extent, they're totally embedded within western culture (the neighbouring suburb of San Bernardino has one of the highest murder rates in the country).

If you plan on checking out *America's own blue zone*, leave your cigarettes at home; it's actually prohibited to even smoke in the city of Loma Linda and, I'm sure sadly for some of you, most people abstain from alcohol as well so you can leave the Californian reds in the car.

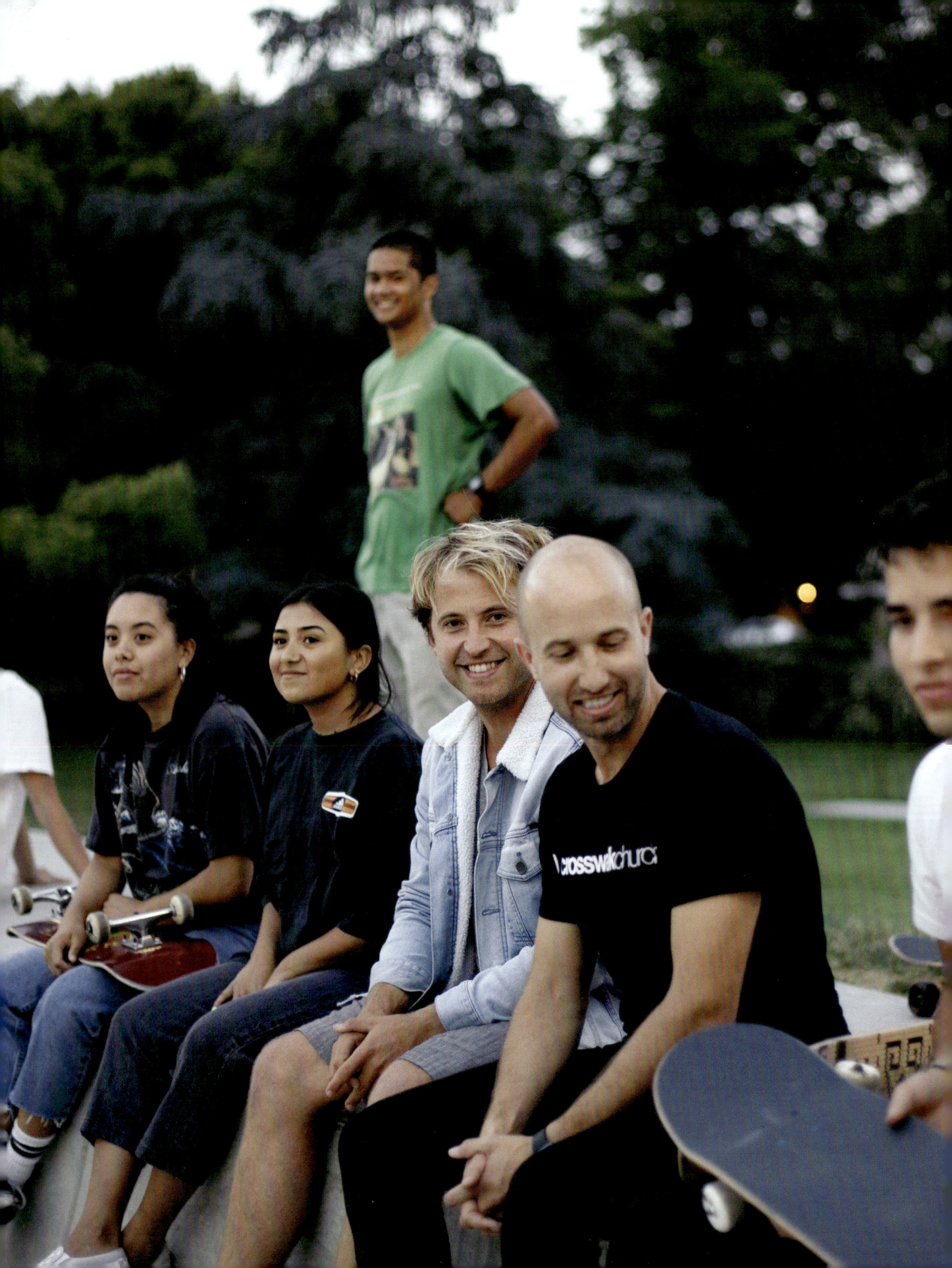

In Loma Linda, men experience 66% less coronary heart disease than their average Californian counterparts, women a whopping 98% less. For stroke, the numbers are equally as impressive, 72% lower for men and 82% lower for women.

Perhaps, after all, one doesn't need to move to a beautiful island paradise to get well and stay well?

Loma Linda is predominately a Seventh-day Adventist community. It is strongly underpinned by this shared faith which drives certain behaviours known to enhance longevity and wellbeing such as a whole foods (often vegetarian) diet and regular exercise.

There is, admittedly, also a heavy influence of western culture here, with conventional burger joints and burrito hubs scattered throughout. However amongst the Seventh-day Adventists there is certainly a modern approach to nutrition and wellbeing; the local organic market is stellar, filled with the best of California produce, and the heavy emphasis on a plant based approach has evolved into an abundance of juices, fermented beverages and kale chips being consumed amongst the people.

It was here in Loma Linda that I experienced such an overwhelming sense of community that I actually felt emotional several times. Attending church for the first time was as equally exciting as it was daunting – notions of the mystical and metaphorical were balanced by such startlingly powerful insights into life that I couldn't help but be quietly impressed.

I was invited to assist in the community outreach program where the church offers a free meal and shower for those in the area who are living on the street. A long line of those who had clearly experienced a tough time in life ran out the door and I struggled to serve lasagne quickly enough alongside the salads already on their plate. As I looked around I was met by a stream of kind, excited smiles from the church volunteers, each scoop of lasagne and salad as nourishing to us emotionally as it was physically for those who hadn't had a meal in days.

Afterward I was gleefully encouraged to join in on a skate session with a dozen of the church members at a nearby skatepark. After a short, embarrassingly poor ride I opted to sit back and observe rather than partake. Mike, our bubbly, energetic contact at the church, a thirty-something pastor with skating ability to envy, rolled casually up to me for a chat.

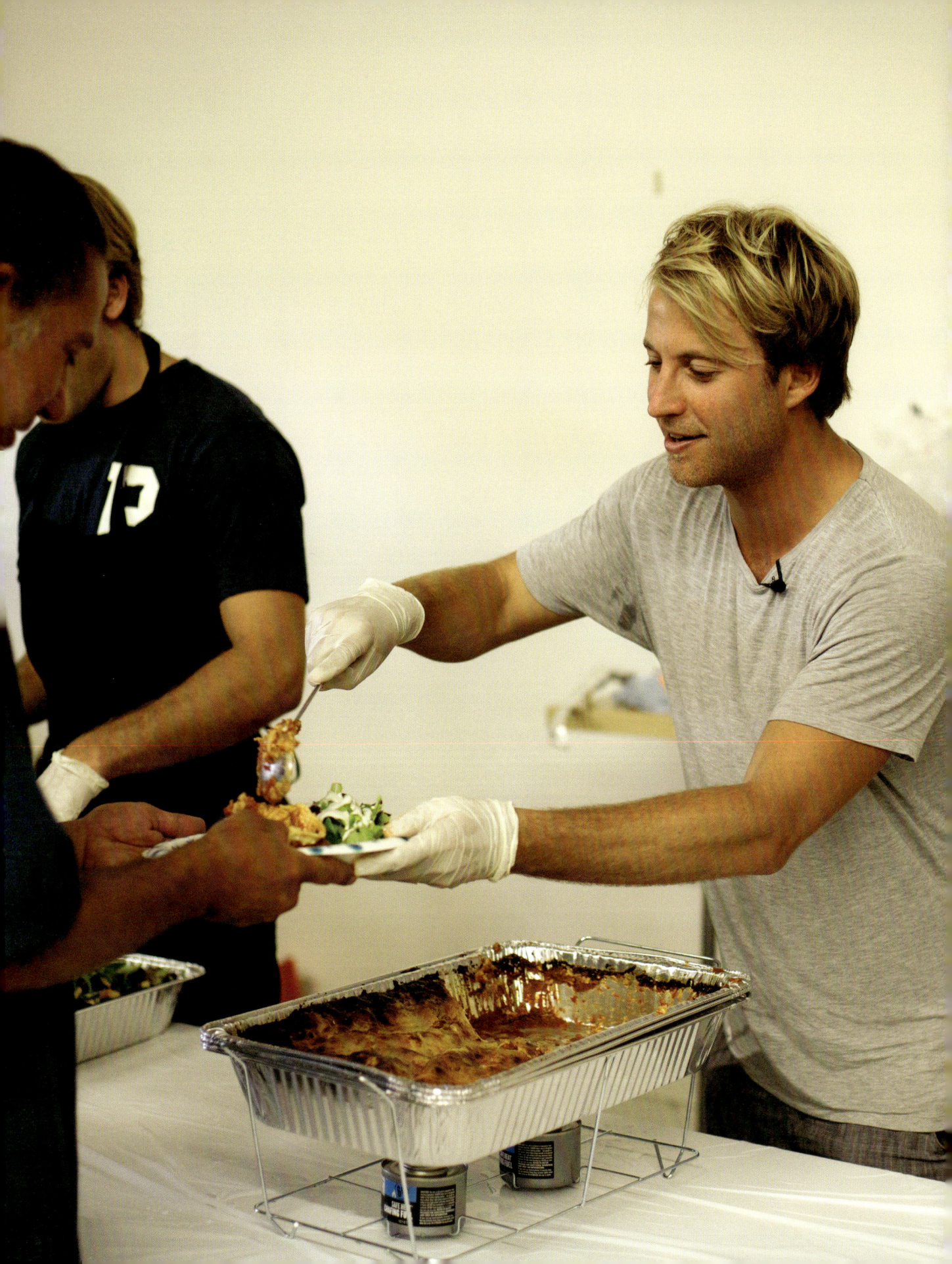

"This is what it's about man. So pumped you're here!"

It's about community for the Seventh-day Adventists. Surrounded by the youth of Loma Linda it was as plain as day that the driving force behind everyone's attendance at the park was to soak up each other's company. Just a thirst for fun, smiles and good times without any interest in talking business, money or other topics often on the table at home. Most of these kids are studying medicine at the local university, their studies include lessons on vegetarianism and wholefoods cooking alongside the medicine component.

"This is the best medicine right here! And surfing!" One said as he perused my Instagram feed.

I smiled, they couldn't be more relatable if they tried
– *is it really this simple?*

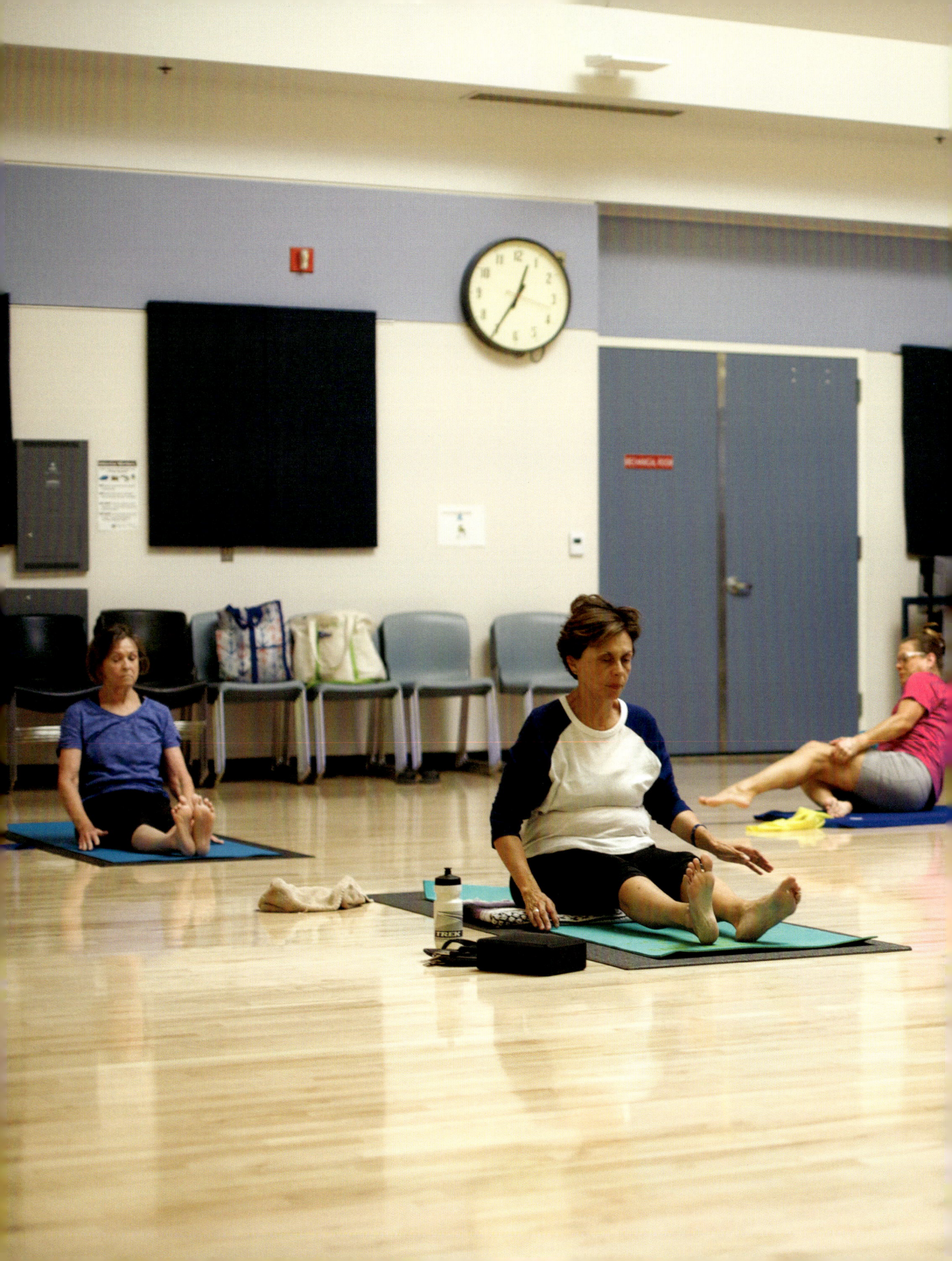

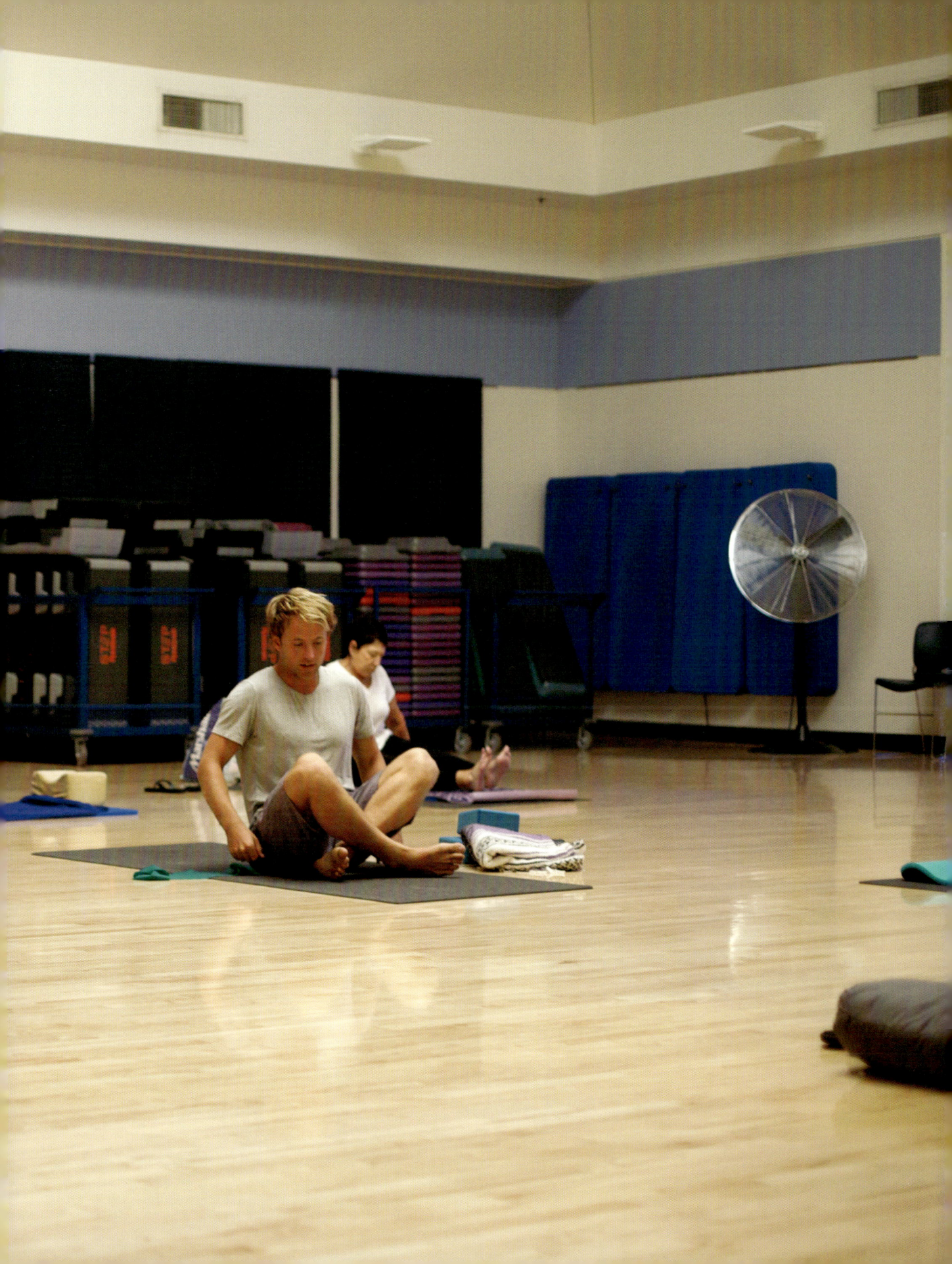

Ikaria, Greece

Flying into Ikaria, a rocky, mountainous island about a 50 minute flight away from Athens, is an experience to remember. Our small, Cessna-like barrel of a plane swayed sideways and rocked back and forth as if performing aerial manoeuvres for a judging panel observing from the short runway below. But there was none. And there was little room for error as we slammed down on the tarmac and began rapidly approaching the end of the runway which spans coast to coast on the island's sun-blasted southern tip.

Aptly named *the island where people forget to die*, Ikarian people are some of the healthiest on the planet. With life expectancies exceeding ours by about 10 years (they reach the age of 90 at 3x the rate at which we do), they also have very little neurodegenerative diseases, depression, heart disease and cancer.

Apparently the baggage handlers were on Ikarian time, we'd been forewarned about this phenomenon, because even though we were the only plane in sight our luggage took about a half hour to appear on the trundling carousel.

Ikaria may be the quintessential longevity culture. A moderately paced, unique Mediterranean lifestyle underpins this Greek island and it's stunning vistas do nothing but put one at peace with the world, the effect enhanced by the jovial smiles one receives from the locals and the charming Greek music played either live or via radio at all the local hang outs.

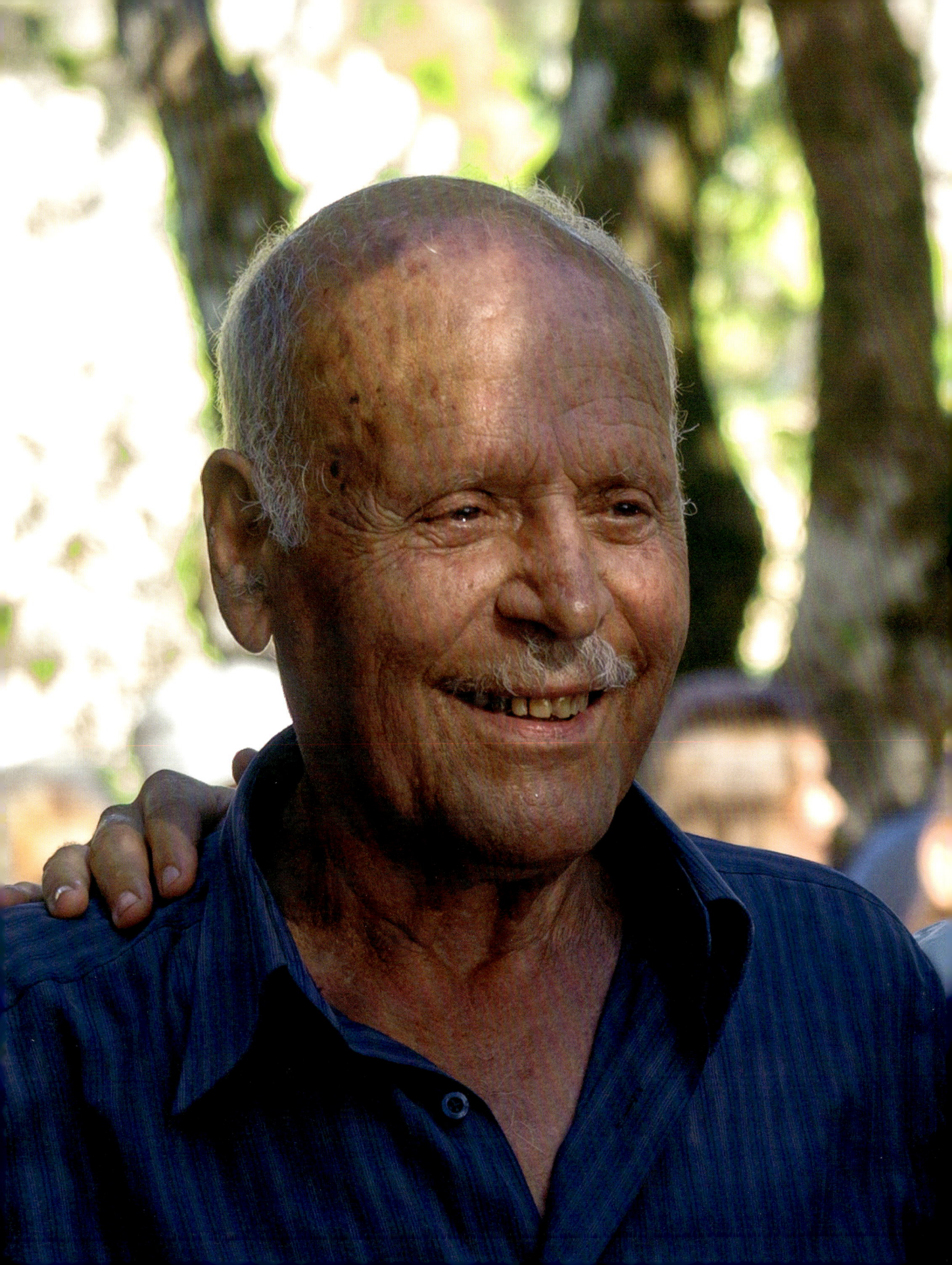

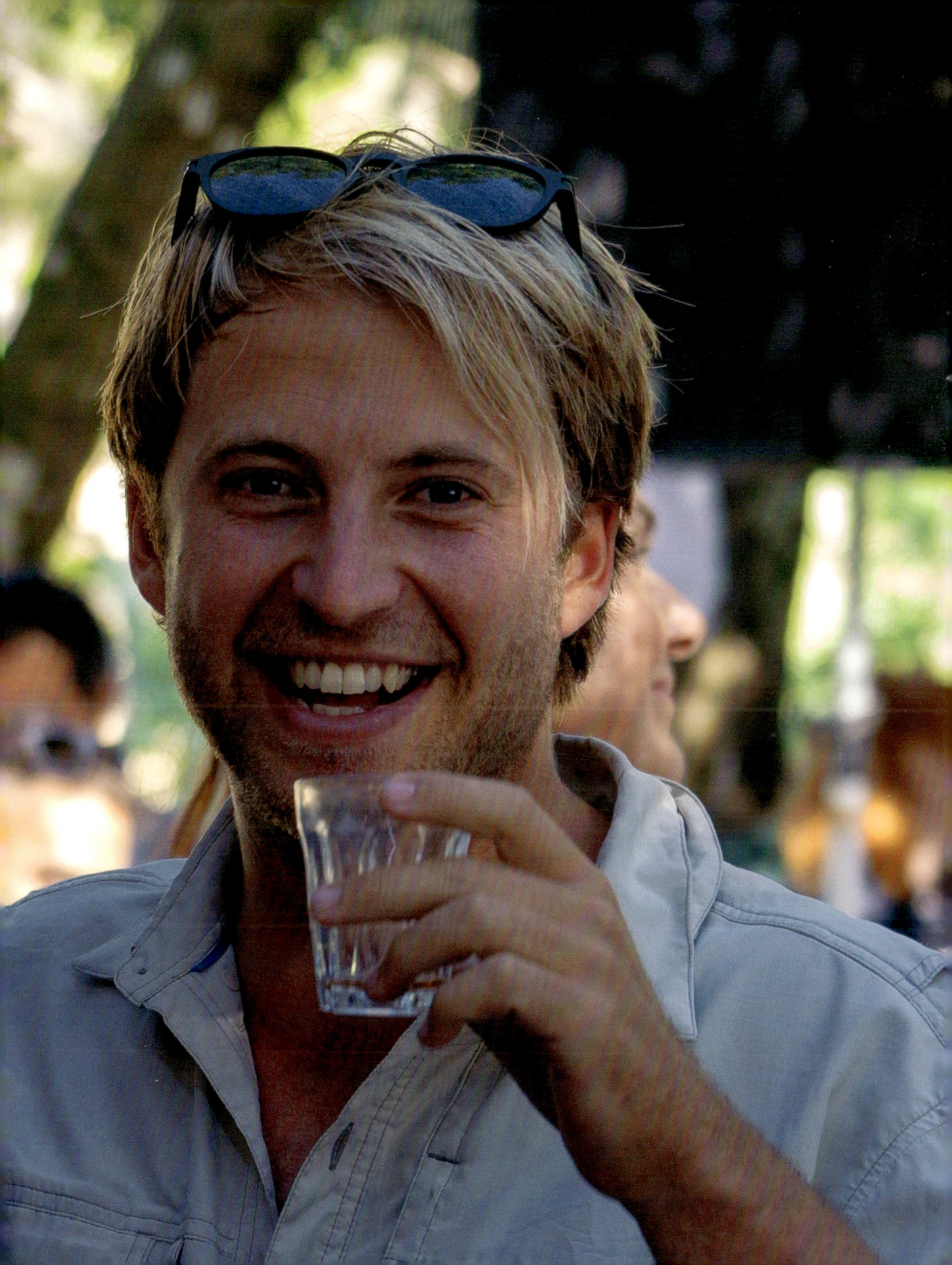

"We're either 200 years ahead or 200 years behind – no one can work it out," Thea, owner of Thea's Inn, the island's go-to accomodation spot, said whilst we chatted over a Greek coffee.

We were invited to meet one of the locals who provided his revered honey to the community, a deeply herbal and dark flavoured food with strong floral elements. George (pronounced Yorigo') is 88 years old. He owns a busy store up in the mountains and we arrived to him instructing numerous forklift drivers to deliver goods around his warehouse. Notably, there seemed to be a deep reverence afforded him by the younger employees and he operated with the sharp alacrity of someone much younger. Upon seeing us he strode over to shake hands.

"Daxo." Okay.

He hopped in my car and rode shotgun, waving dismissively at the seatbelt alert as it pinged incessantly.

"It's for your seatbelt," I motioned.

"Eh. Psh." Not interested.

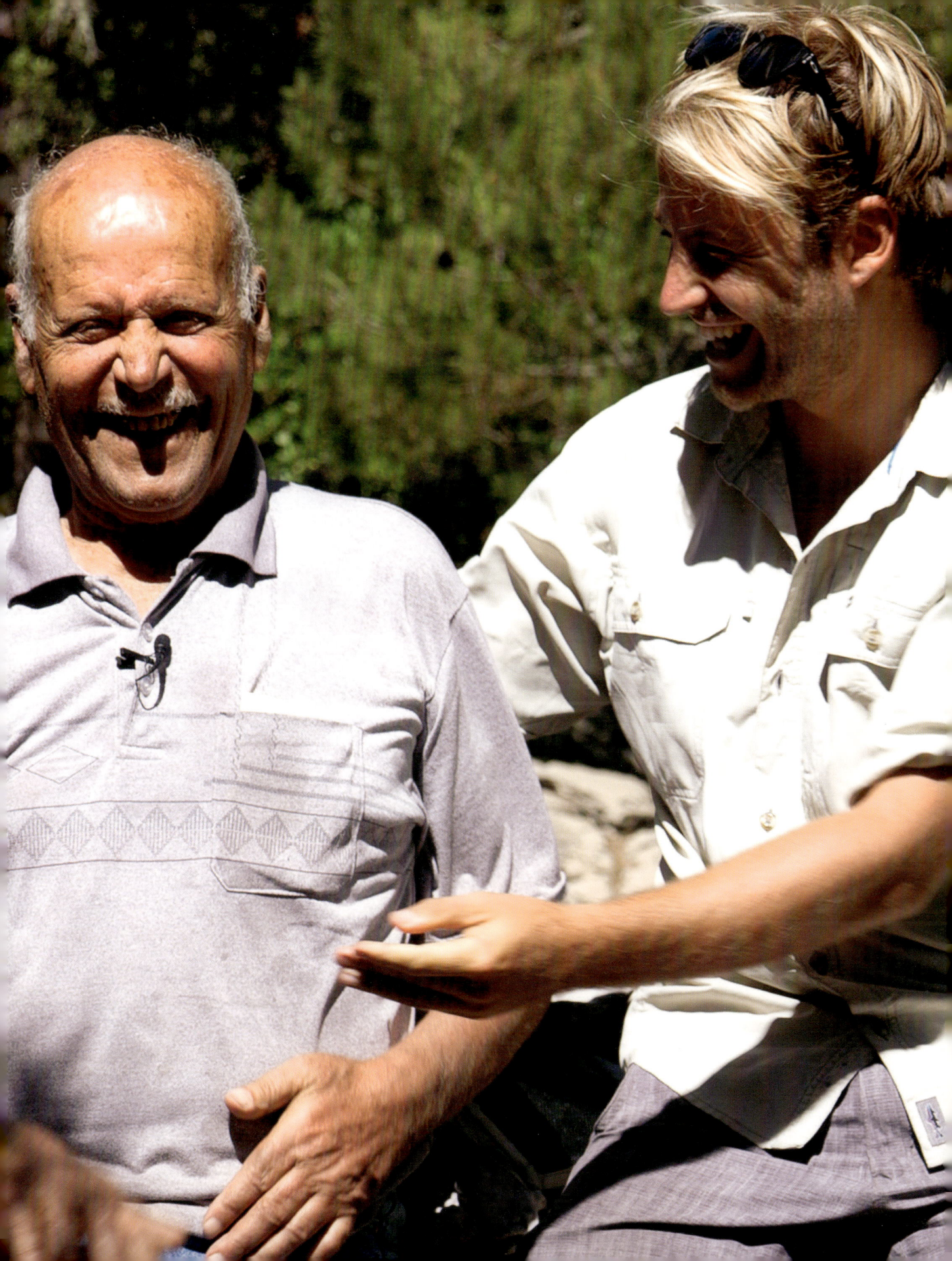

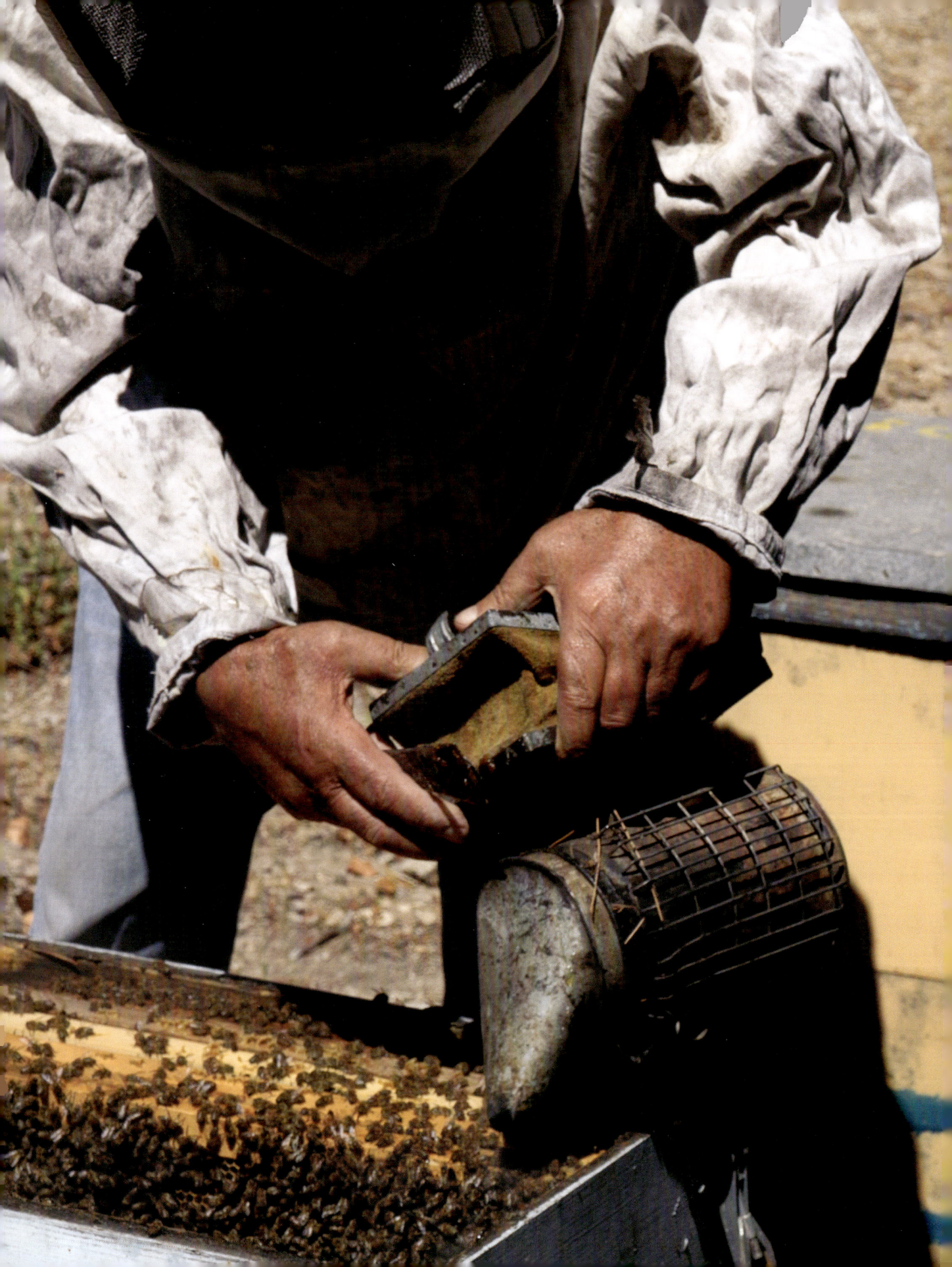

We arrived at the large network of hives George keeps further up in the wilderness and we all climbed into bee suits. He proceeded to show me his wild organic honey operation and persisted through several stings, cursing in Greek each time as he pumped more smoke onto the buzzing hive. One of the bees found its way inside my suit and decided to investigate my inner ear. It took everything not to slash and swipe at it but eventually it left me alone – after it did I informed George.

"It was seeing if you good or bad," he said. "No sting? You good maybe."

I asked him how he's so busy and fit at 88, after all, he is 8 years older than the average male life expectancy in Australia and most at his age have retired to a largely inactive lifestyle.

"You must keep moving. And be busy. Everything in moderation. You can't enjoy rest if you're not tired."

My preconceived notions of Ikarian culture being a slow-motion lackadaisical lifestyle were shattered as I watched the elder community adopt their roles in society. They worked hard, very hard.

In Ikaria, they say *a man is nothing if he does not have olives and a vineyard.*

All of the elderly people I met and spoke with had formidable sized gardens to which they tended every single day, often climbing up steep steps, jumping through fences and squatting low to care for. I toured Illias Parikos' (Thea's husband's) two gardens for hours and could barely keep up with his sharp wit and quick movement around the property. Illias is used to being interviewed, it seemed, as he reeled off a list of production companies who'd also come to the farm to film.

"Ah, so you're famous." I offered.

"Yes. Maybe I go Hollywood soon." He barely smirked.

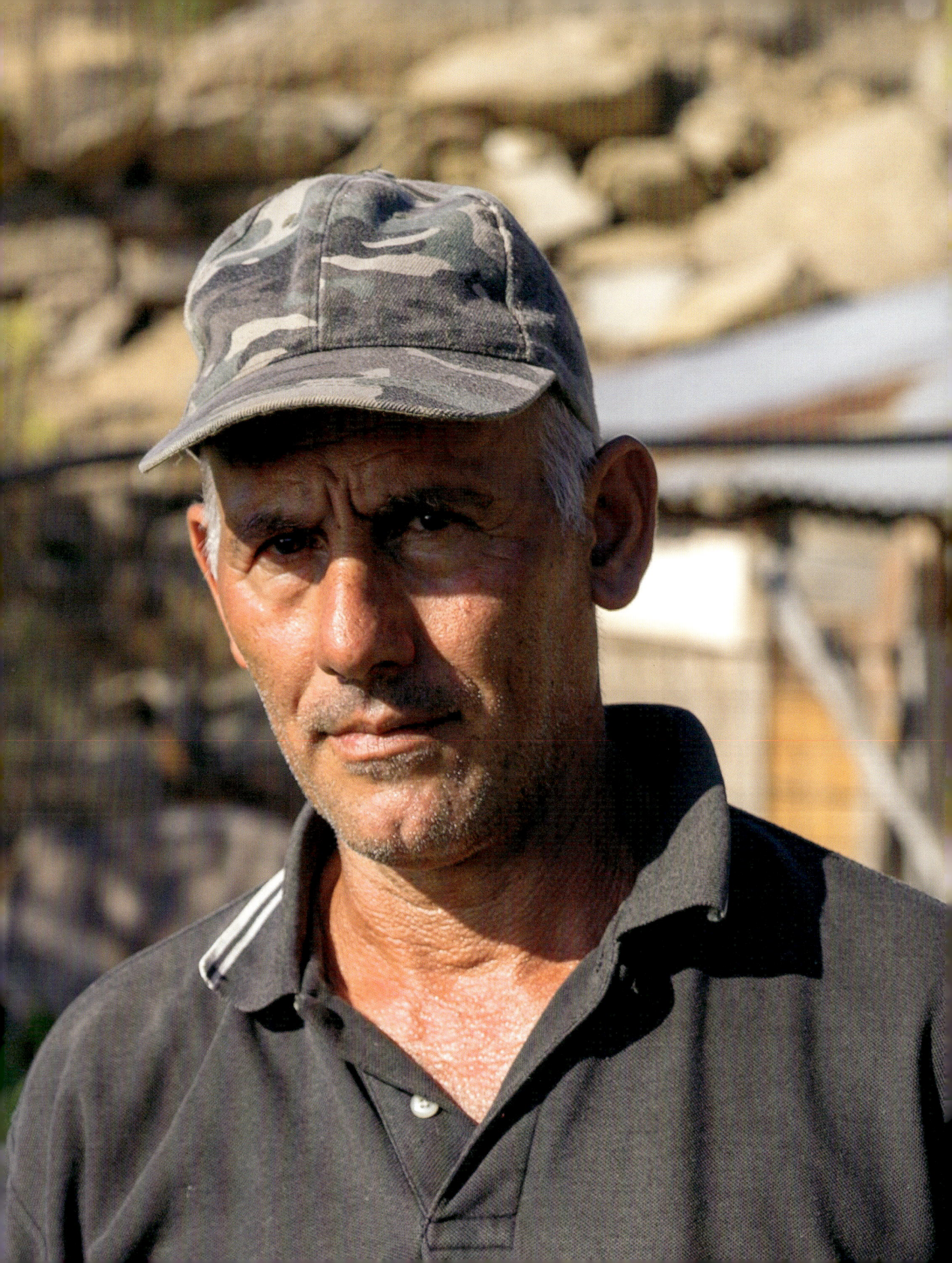

Illias' garden provides for the family but also most of the food on the restaurant's menu. There is a plethora of strawberries on offer, many of which I hungrily jammed into my mouth before he admonished me lightheartedly.

"No. Stop eating. We make daiquiris later. If someone like you comes every day we are finished." He grins widely and chuckles, his youthful face glowing in the hot, dry afternoon sun as it sparkles over the mediterranean ocean down the cliff below.

At the end of a 12 hour work day, Illias is often busy grilling lamb or goat in the kitchen at the restaurant, uncomplaining and with a big smile on his face. There is no stress, no urgency, just a stoic and persistent enjoyment in the work as if *there is no other place to be besides in that very moment.*

Your own longevity lifestyle

This book is intended to be read whilst sitting back on a comfy couch, basking in some delicious winter sunshine and sipping your favourite morning drink.

My intention with this book is to inspire you into action, or inaction in many cases. To inspire you to take back control of your time and to spend it on the things which matter to you. Those valuable activities in your life also turn out to be the most nourishing. As nourishing, at least, as those delicious and colourful meals you choose to eat every day.

This book might be about *longevity*, but it is also about *wellness*. Wellness should exist throughout life from a very young age to a very old age. We begin to think about ageing when we start getting sick at middle age, however we should not separate this from the health experiences we have in our younger years, too. Following the lifestyle of the longevity cultures ensures not only a *long* life, but also a *good* life.

This means that it is never too early, or too late, to start putting these ideas into practice.

So, sit back, relax and, piece by piece, let's learn about the *four pillars of longevity & wellness.*

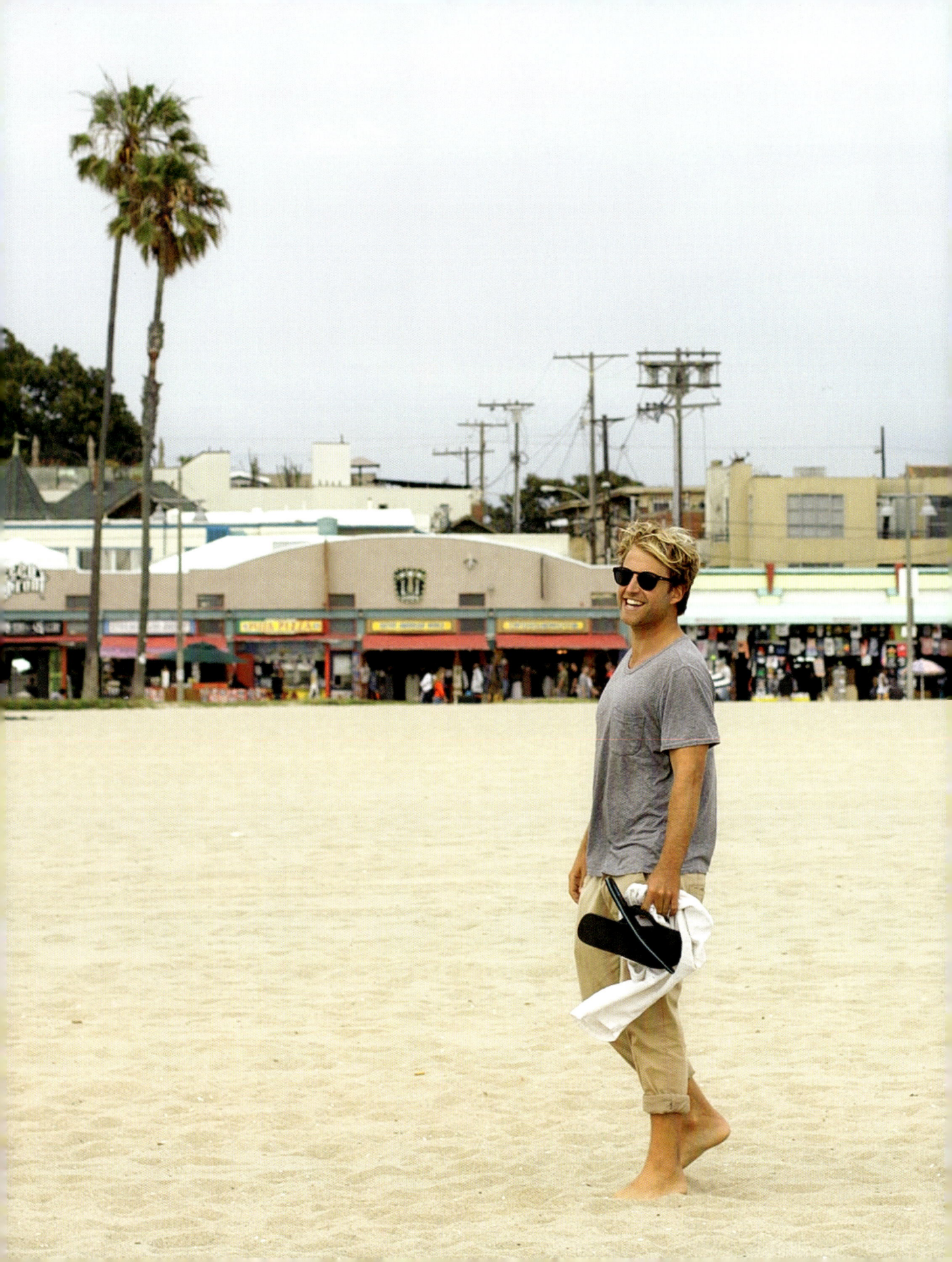

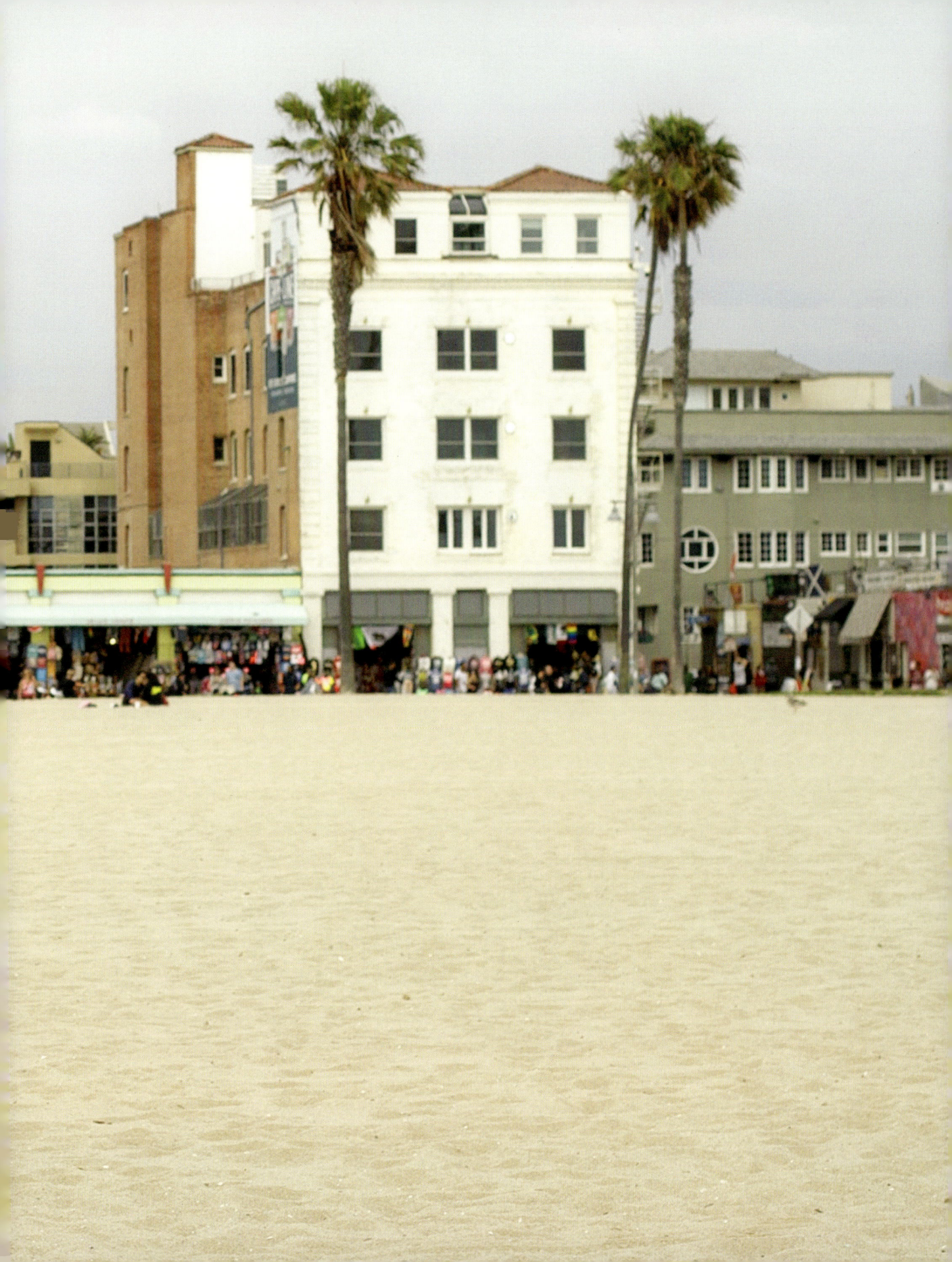

_____ Nutrition

"You can't make chicken salad out of chicken shit. You eat garbage, you're guna' make garbage."

-Paul Chek, renowned trainer & spiritual teacher

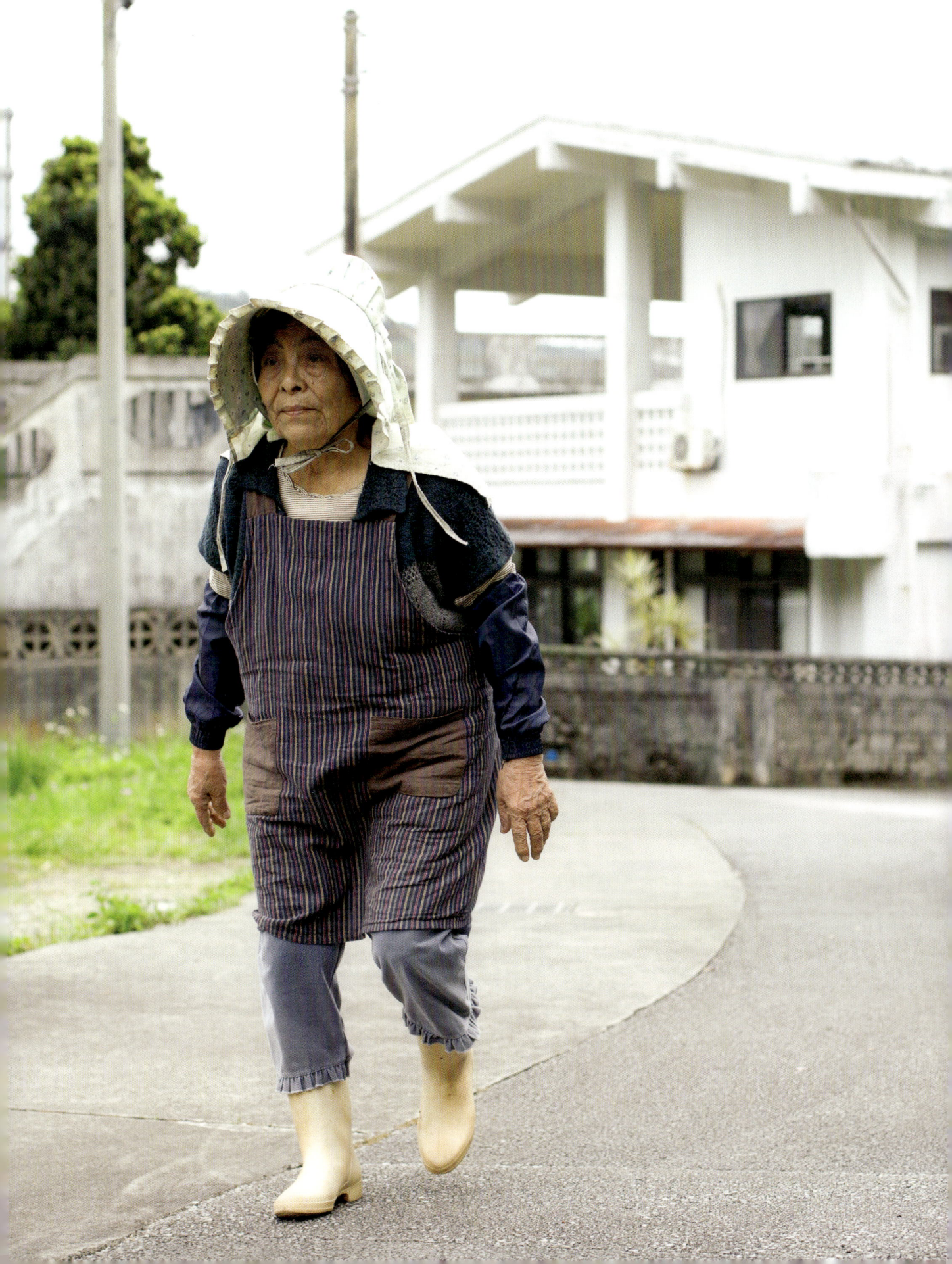

Okinawa,
Japan

Misako Taira, 88, represents an age only 4 years over the average female lifespan in Australia, however she moves with the alacrity and nimbleness of someone decades younger.

Misako can full squat down to her heels or rest with her knees folded beneath her easily. She smiles from this position as we enter her traditional-looking Japanese home at the bottom of a lush gorge of dense, green forest. She's partly watching the television and partly fixing up a piece of clothing, her dexterous hands nipping in and out of the material with a needle and thread. I ask her to mute the television for copyright reasons and she yelps in agreement, popping up like a spring chicken to grab the remote. She has a big smile and is happy to see us.

"What do you want me to do?" She asks, as if an actress who's just stepped on set.

I ask if she'll do some gardening for us and she complains about a local wild boar which persistently steals her favourite vegetables.

"We normally get ten kilos of Okinawan sweet potato per haul but now it is only 3kg because of the boar."

We make our way outside, Misako walking with a slight limp but no other outward sign of physical hindrance. Her garden is five metres from her front door and edges onto the street. The light coloured dirt is thick and loamy, the result of countless years of careful tending.

"I will pull these weeds for you," Misako says as she bends down easily, picks up a small pick and begins pulling away at some persistent growth beside her patch of onions.

For Okinawans, and the majority of the longevity cultures, having a fruitful garden means having a *fruitful life*. For many of the people in these cultures, they could not exist without a garden simply because such a large portion of their diet depends on them.

Whether it's a spacious farming operation in Ikaria, Greece or this ten metre squared plot on Misako's property in Okinawa, it is a mark of pride, of self-sufficiency for someone to grow their own food in longevity cultures. The long-lasting tradition of providing for one's self and family through this means is deeply embedded in their lifestyle. Not only is it economically valued, it is also valued as an important tool for health.

"This is the freshest food you can get. I know where it comes from, this is important to me. It is good for me."

Misako is standing patiently whilst I interview her about her garden.

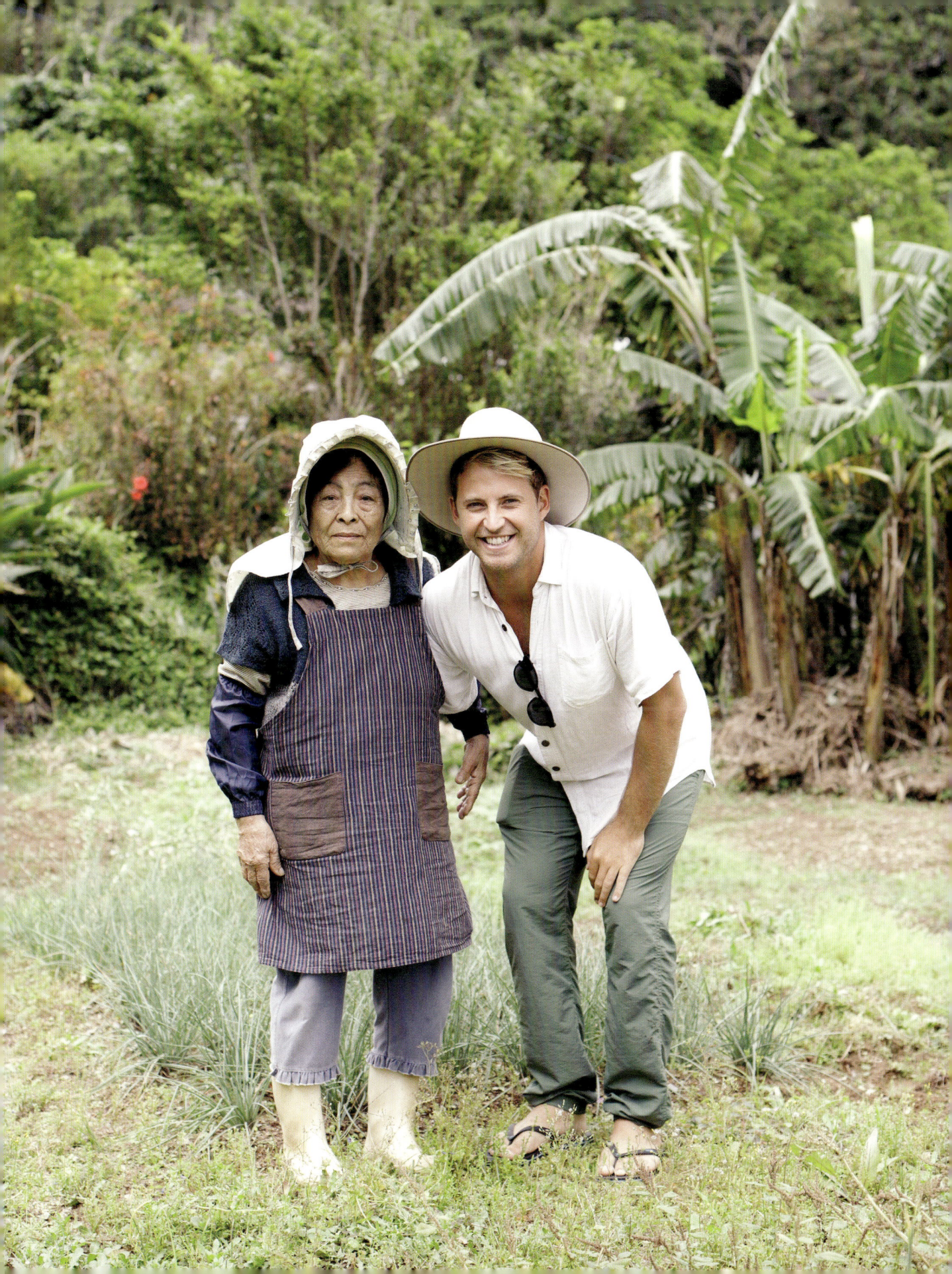

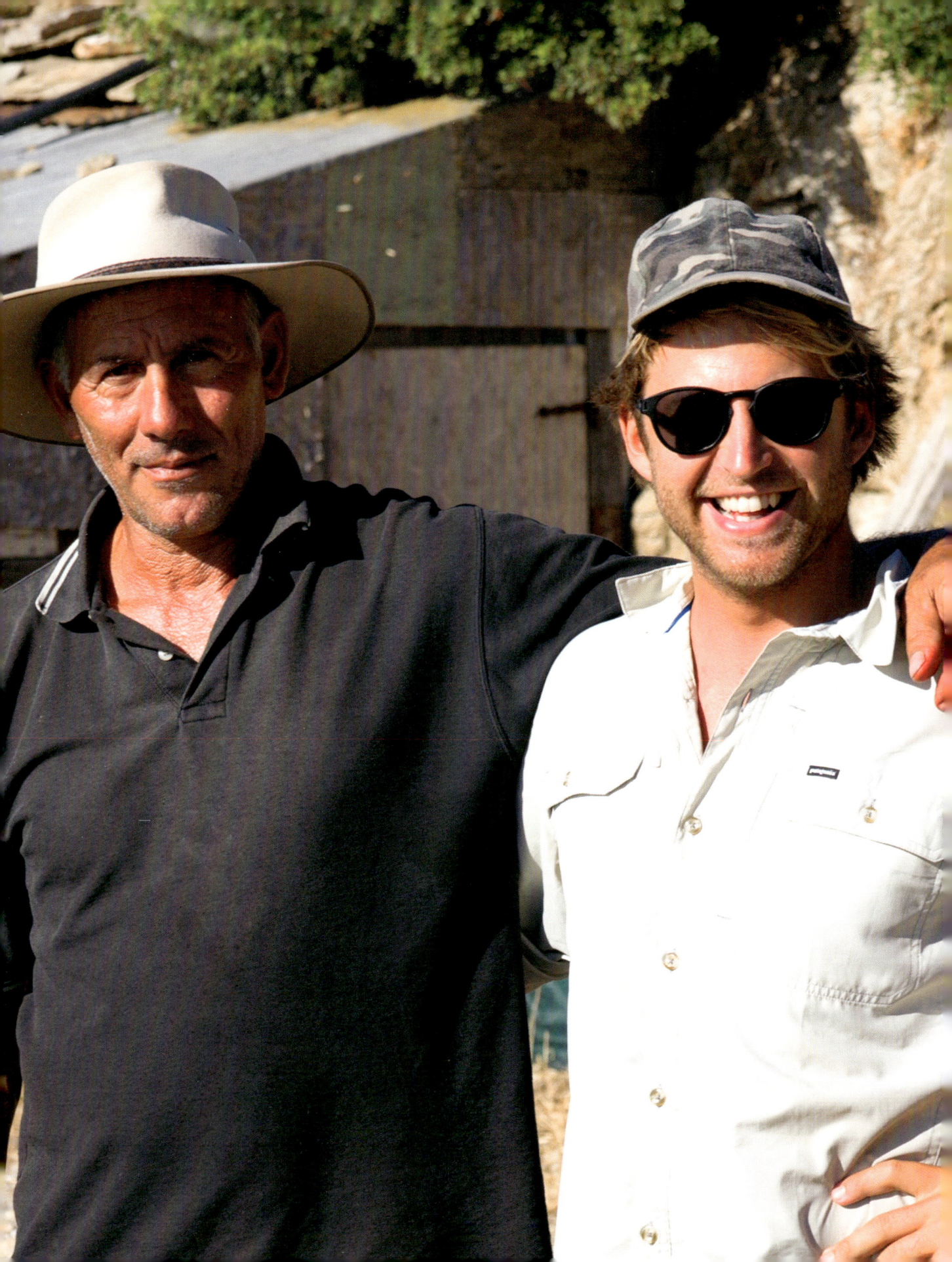

"Do you use chemicals on the garden?"

"No."

"Why?"

"I don't like them, I never have. We have to eat the food so it shouldn't have chemicals on it."

This sentiment was echoed in Ikaria, too. I worked alongside Illeas on his small-scale farming operations where thick groves of citrus burst forth alongside goats, chickens, wild herbs which spring up in their own display of independence against the harsh climate and finally the staple Mediterranean products like tomato, onion, zucchini and cucumber.

I asked Illias if he used chemicals to which I received a passionate response.

"We feed these foods to our children. We don't want to feed chemicals to them. It is not safe," He shares whilst gazing out over the ocean gathering his thoughts.

"It would be easier for us to use the chemicals perhaps. It is not easy to grow here; it is hot and there isn't much water, but because we care so much for the land, and because food is so important to us and our families, we do not use chemicals."

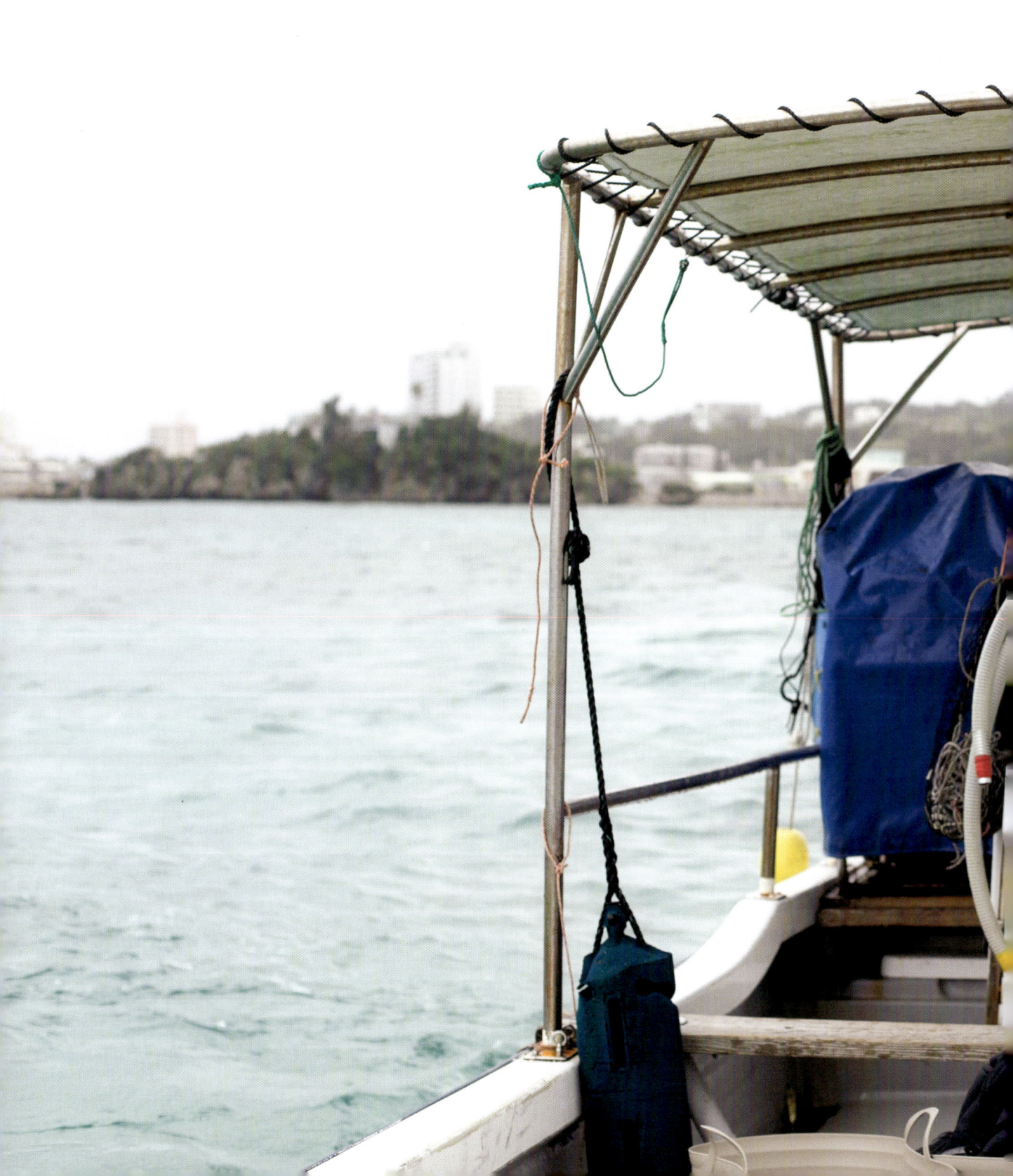

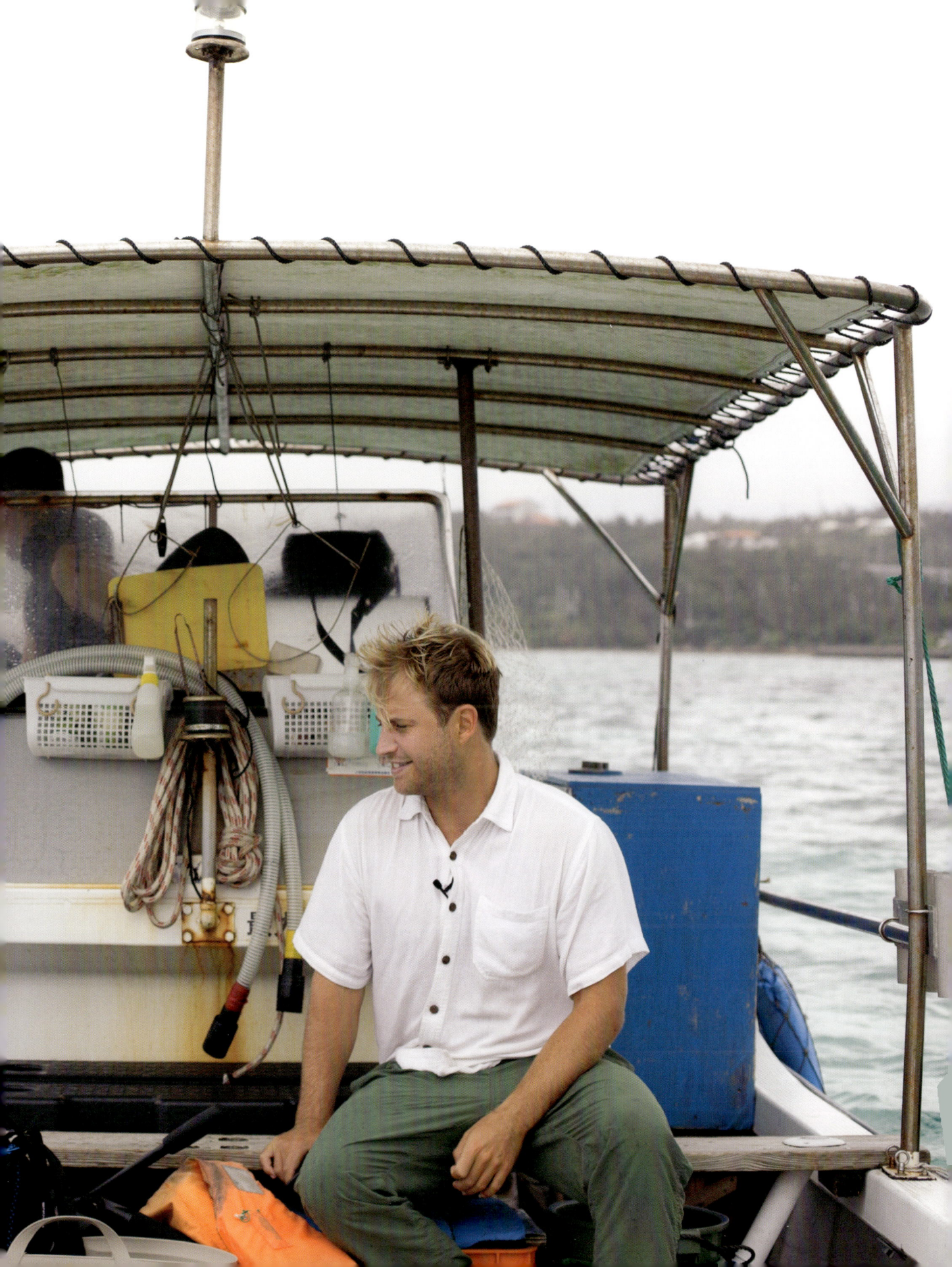

One would also find, if attending other longevity cultures such as Sardinia and the Nicoya Peninsula, that these people also grow the majority of their own food without chemical intervention. The emphasis on an organic, Seasonal, Local, Organic & Wholefoods (SLOW) diet is difficult to miss amongst longevity cultures.

Adopting a fantastic diet like that of the longevity cultures, a stack of plant food alongside more moderate amounts of animal foods, ensures we have great *quality* in our days as well as quantity. If all disease results from inflammation, then we need to live an anti-inflammatory lifestyle, and that starts with the diet.

And the science tends to support this too. When I was in Okinawa I was lucky enough to speak to Dr. Craig Wilcox who shared information about how our diet can *up-regulate* certain longevity genes to better express health.

"One of those longevity genes is FOX 03. FOX 03 reduces inflammation which, at the cellular level, helps to drive the ageing process. You want to live an anti-inflammatory lifestyle, you want a supercharged FOX 03. You can do that through dietary means, such as eating lots of seaweed which contains astaxanthin."

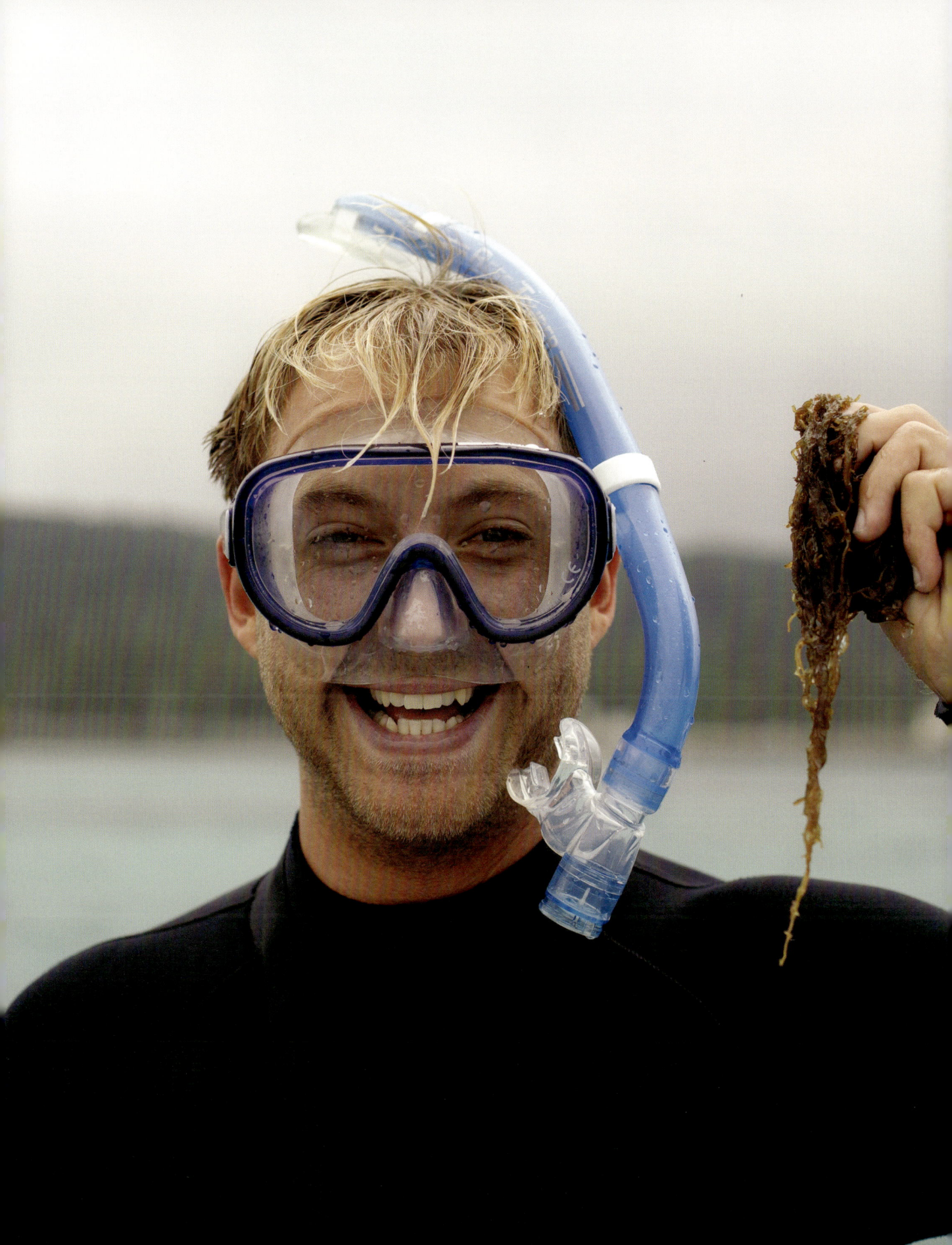

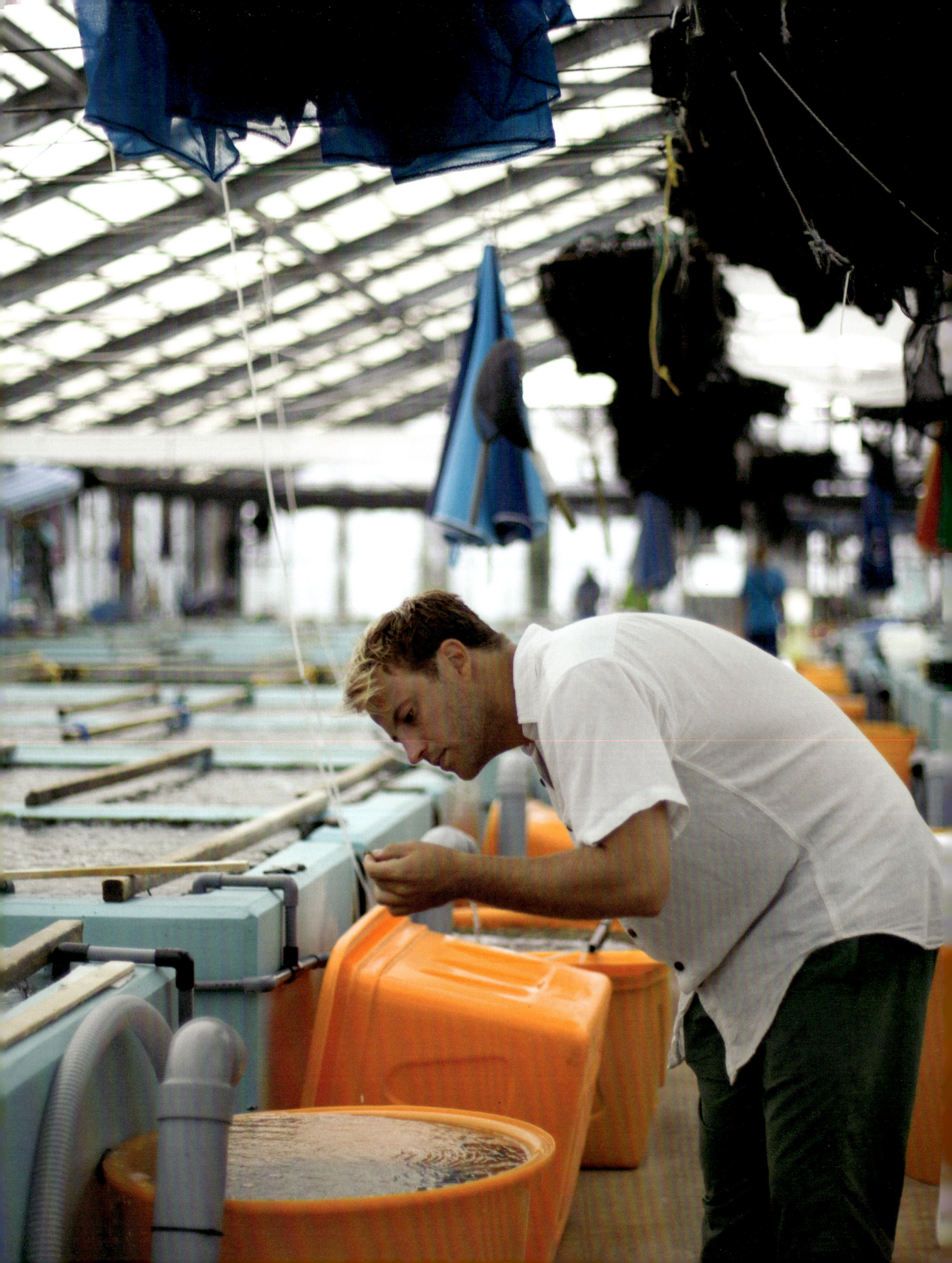

In Okinawa, seaweed is a staple vegetable. I was invited to go and harvest some myself from the local farming operation on the island. Underneath the pristine waters of the surrounding ocean lie fields upon fields of ecologically friendly agriculture where a particular species of seaweed called *mozuku* is grown. Divers swim down to harvest this *mozuku* with a vacuum which sucks the growth off of a crossed network of strings. This is pumped up to a boat on the surface where any superfluous objects are taken out before being sent back to a factory for rinsing and sorting.

Seaweed is a longevity superfood containing an array of fibres, protein and micronutrients (like astaxanthin - a powerful antioxidant) which support optimal functioning of the human body. It is also an ecological miracle and could provide very tangible solutions to our current climate crisis as it sequesters large amounts of carbon from the atmosphere.

"Mozuku is a fast food here," Dr. Wilcox says, sitting aside his desk at the university in Okinawa. "You can run down to the local store, buy a packet, tear the top off and eat it straight. A longevity super snack."

The longevity cultures are not extreme in the way they eat. In fact, in every sense of the word, they are moderate because they tend to consume a little bit of everything. In recent times, some longevity researchers have suggested that these cultures are strictly plant-based, but based on my observations this is untrue.

In Okinawa, fish is a staple part of the diet and traditionally made up a significant portion of people's caloric intake. In Ikaria, wild goat is consumed with gusto but mostly at celebratory events such as a panagiri. In Loma Linda, where people are mostly Seventh Day Adventists, a vegetarian or pescatarian diet is followed meaning small amounts of animal foods are still present.

Indeed, if we were to analyse all of the longevity cultures, we would find that they follow, to a large extent, a seasonal, local, organic & whole foods diet with no heavy emphasis on restriction of any food group (with the exception of Loma Linda in their vegetarianism). We would also find that they enjoy growing their own food which offers a cascade of health benefits such as movement, sunshine & meditative practice. And finally, we find that they often eat until they are 80% full - this is easily achieved in such environments because they often eat amidst conversation with friends or family which naturally slows down consumption.

"Eat food. Not too much, mostly plants."

-Michael Pollan, world-renowned researcher & author

These are some helpful ideas for you to start to appropriate an excellent nutritional regiment in your life.

Listen to your body

Your own inner nutritionist will tell you the foods it needs. Operate from a basis of *did it grow in the ground once? Did it run around or swim around once? And have they done much to it since?* Limit your food choices based off of those questions and refine from there.

Start a garden

Growing your own will mean you have the freshest produce possible which offers up a plethora of phytonutrient potential (anti-ageing!). You'll also be able to ensure an organic operation, limit yourself to seasonal produce and give yourself the benefit of some sunshine and natural movement, too.

Shop at farmers markets

Shopping at farmer's markets develops a relationship with your food providers. It also ensures you eat seasonally, locally and (hopefully) organically.

Do more share platters

Enjoying great food with friends slows down consumption, adds the benefit of great conversation and anchors food to a healthy activity. In the longevity cultures, food is used to bring people together.

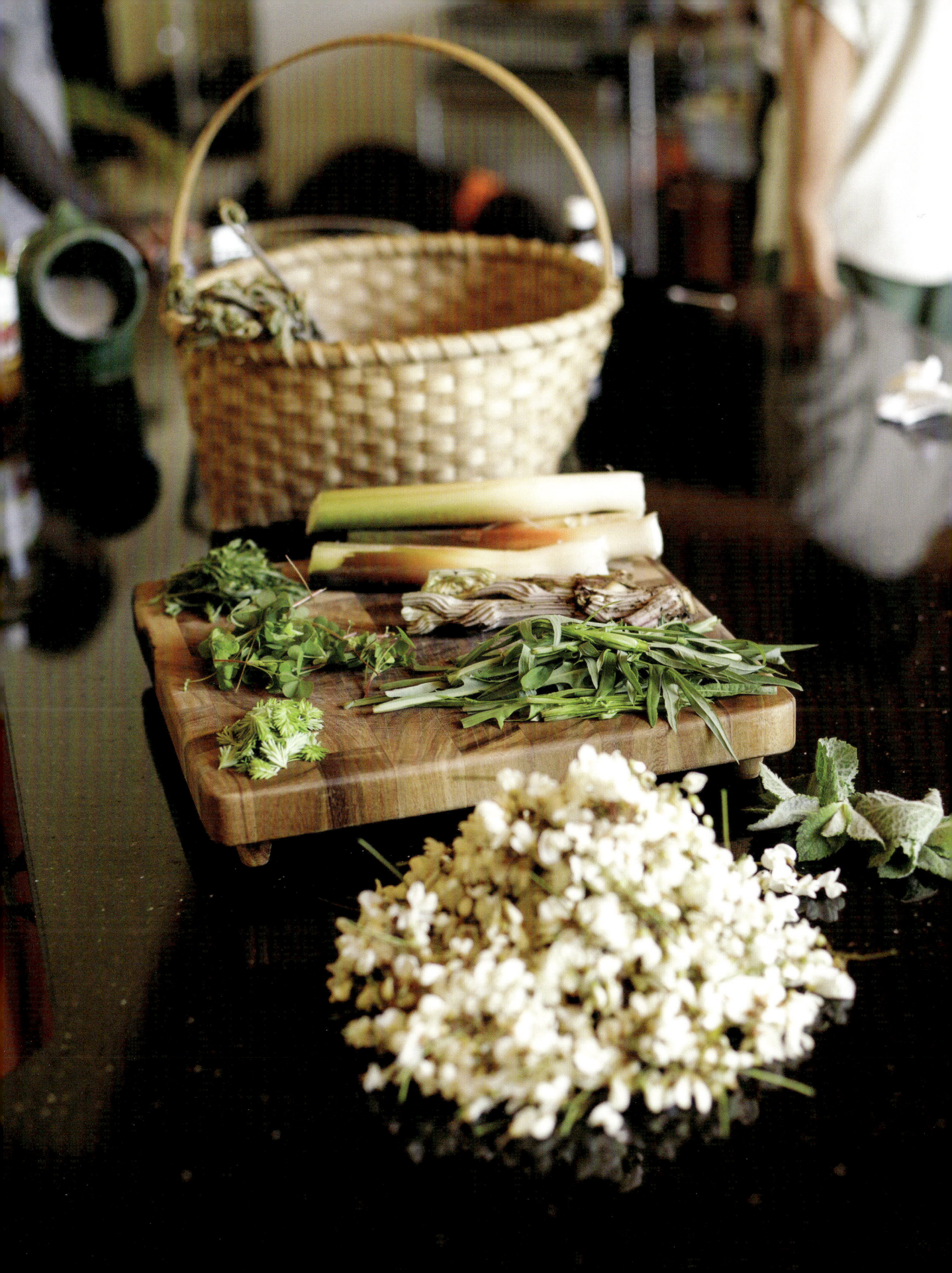

Food for thought...

Could wine be a part of longevity?

Whether it's the lightly coloured, naturally fermented home-made red wine of Ikaria or the dark, dry Grenache red in Sardinia, when it comes to the observation of cultures who live a long time – one may come to the conclusion that alcohol, in particular, wine, *may actually contribute* to their longevity.

Ikaria, Greece

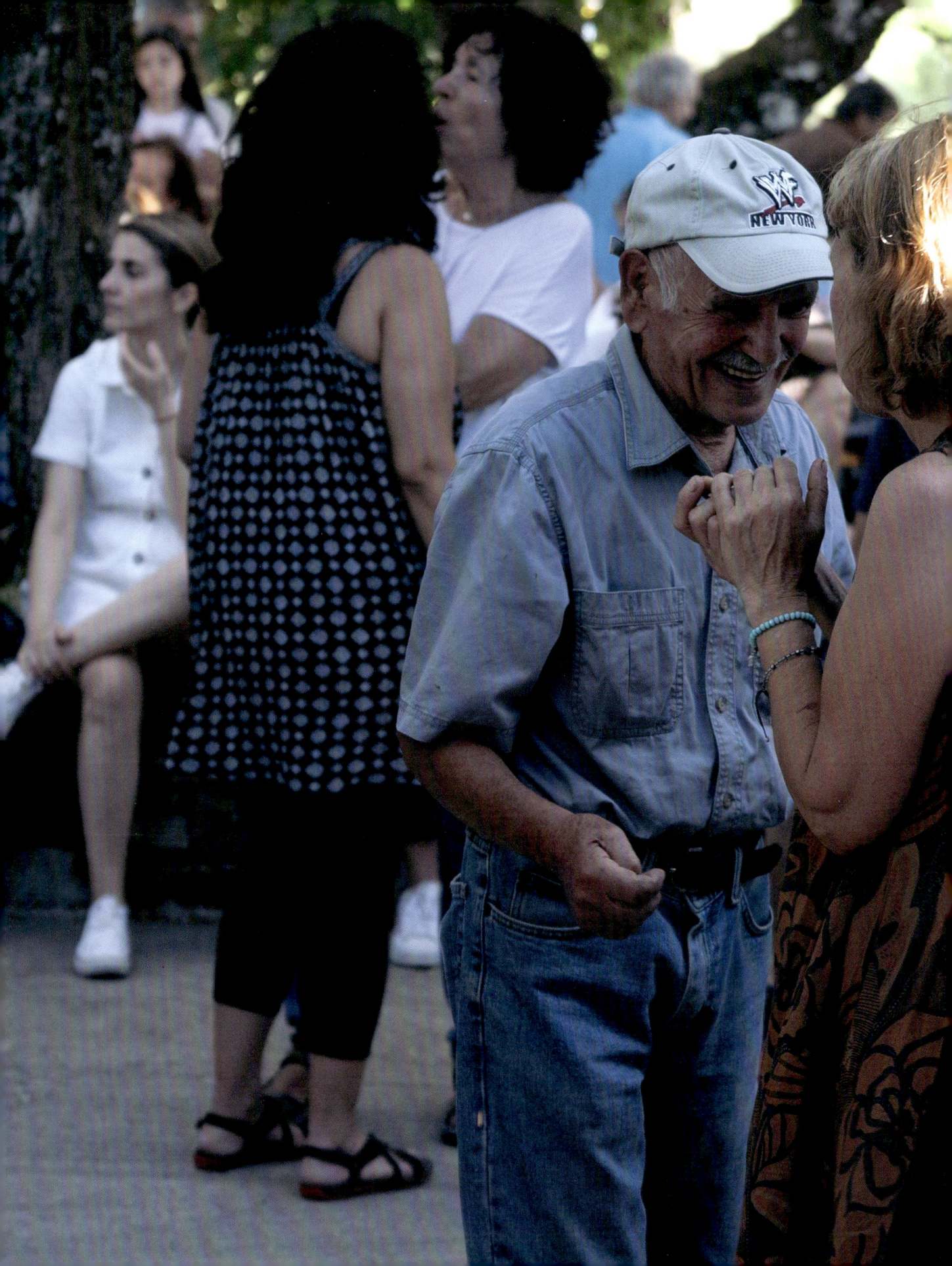

"It's ten in the morning and the wine tastes like it's been spiked with vodka."

I took a final gulp of the light, cherry-coloured red swirling in a small glass in my hand. Indeed, it seemed to taste better with every sip, the harsh bite fading away into a sweet and fermented after taste.

"We'd better start dancing soon I hope." I added, feeling slightly buzzed already and somewhat self conscious of just how much *buzz* the camera would be picking up from across the table.

It was in fact, ten in the morning. And this was a new feat for me. I could hardly believe that I was drinking wine, eating bread and slow cooked goat on an island in the Aegean Sea which has been assigned the tag line; *the island where people forget to die.*

The people in Ikaria have extreme wellbeing. I was here to find out just how they were achieving such feats.

Are they meditating and doing yoga? They're surely fasting! I concluded.

"You must eat now!" Our on-the-ground contact in Ikaria, Eleni, interrupted my thoughts. "Every time you drink, you must eat." She motioned to a plate of Greek salad (all homegrown) and goat.

"I'm so full already."

"*Daxo.* Okay. So you move around a bit then you come back and eat."

I was attending an Ikarian *Panagiri*. A religious celebration up in a dry, rocky, mountainous village of the island. This was, apparently, the best panagiri you could hope to attend because it was the *true, authentic* expression of Ikarian culture.

A thousand year old church stood in the middle of a large, tiled courtyard, a small kitchen had been built nearby out of beautiful sandstone and would act as the service area for the hundreds of people due to attend the event later that day. All the while the blistering sun did its best to penetrate the thick branches offering a natural shelter for the area which would eventually turn into a dance floor 8 hours later.

It was all very Mediterranean.

I watched as a small lorry backed into the courtyard carrying dozens upon dozens of bottles of local Ikarian red wine. Eleni informs me it is all home-made, organic & preservative free.

"It is real wine. You never tasted anything like it."

I certainly hadn't. *Nor had I consumed so much before lunch time*, I mused. I was recruited to help lift the heavy crates off the back of the truck and deliver them into the kitchen area. They were stacked, crate upon crate, behind a counter which people would approach, buy a wine followed by goat & salad, and take it out to their table to consume amongst friends and family. The money collected would be distributed amongst the local village as the local people saw fit.

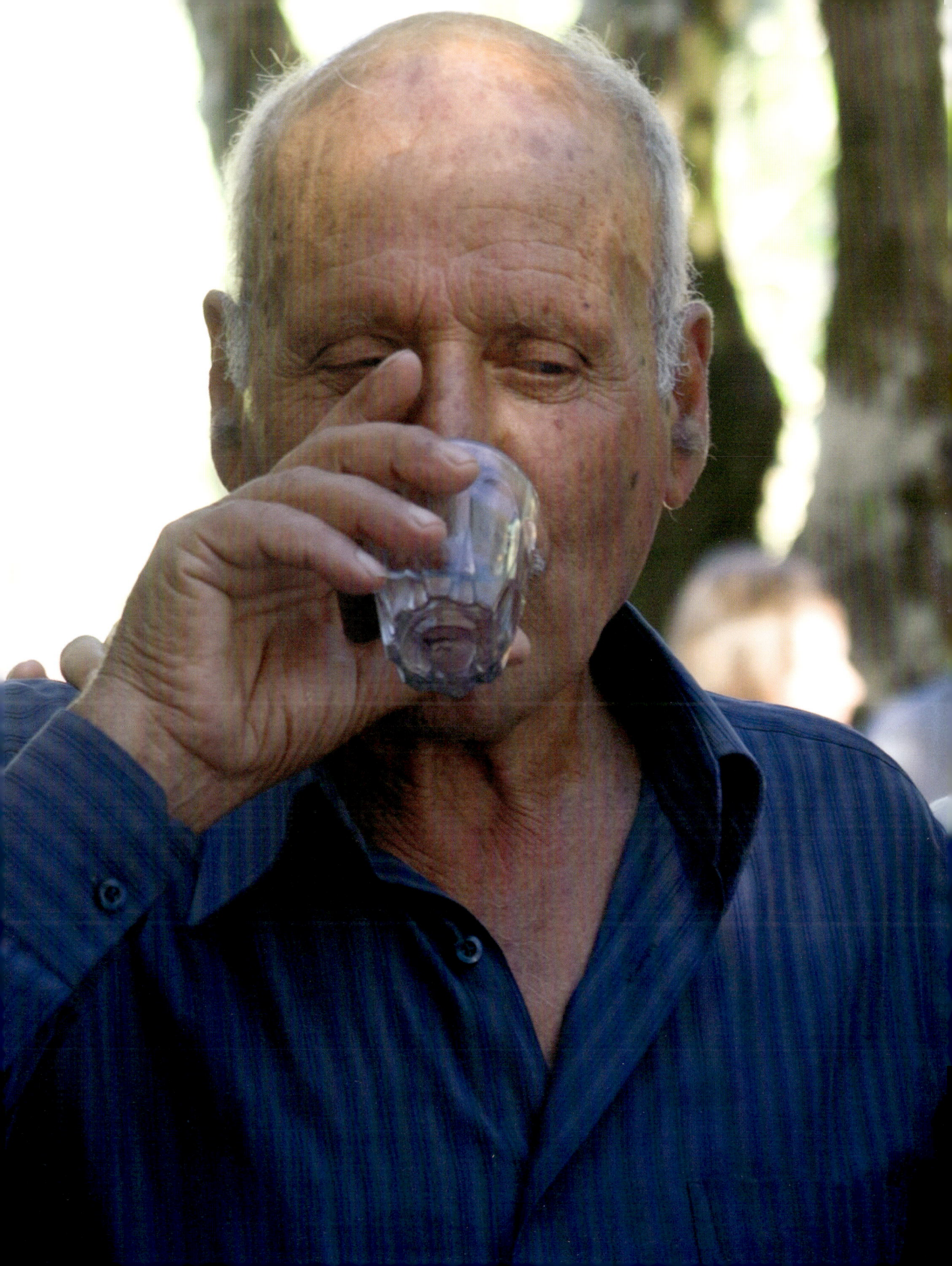

Sure, there's research out there supporting the health benefits of certain wines, in particular red wine (Grenache in particular), such as reduced risk for cardiovascular disease, but in my opinion none of these studies were really solid. I knew that antioxidants, like those found in red wine, reduce inflammation and that ageing and disease are rooted in inflammation. But it was difficult to quantify if wine or alcohol was good or bad. *It would be left up to observation*, I thought.

"The wine is a big part of your culture, then?" I asked Eleni.

"Yes. But it's more than that. It's about what the wine represents; what it does. For instance you never drink alone in Ikaria. Always with friends or family. It is used to bring people together for conversation, dancing and food."

Thea Parikos, the owner of Thea's Inn, a beautiful accomodation space back down the mountain chimes in. "You'll very rarely see someone get drunk here. It's frowned upon to get drunk in Ikaria. The wine is used as a social lubricant of sorts. It gets people talking and dancing and having fun."

I thought back to the notes I had taken about the two previous locations I had visited. It seemed, and this was certainly backed by the research, that community & social ties were one of, if not *the most* important factor in determining the longevity & quality of one's life.

In Okinawa I had visited a saké factory and attended Moari meetings where the men, in particular, enjoyed plenty of it. I had watched a 93 year old down a frothy beer with her mates then go sing 6 karaoke songs after spending all day dancing. I had heard about groups of shepherds in Sardinia carrying large containers of Grenache with them all day whilst working the fields and sharing them over lunch. But I hadn't thought about the *side effects* of the alcohol in this way, the *indirect* benefits of **how & who** *the alcohol was consumed with.*

What I was seeing in front of me was this beautiful display of alcohol being used intelligently. Not to get drunk, but to limit one's inhibitions, not to blunt emotions, but to liberate them into friendly discussion and importantly to enhance the strong undercurrent of presence, relaxation and fun which was so tangible at this celebration.

I wondered how I would convey this revelation to the people watching my film or reading my work back home. How could I disentangle what I thought to be the misconstrued notion that all alcohol is the same? Because if anything, these cultures were consuming the premium version of it, the organic, preservative free versions – surely that was important? They consumed the alcohol most often with food and didn't drink excessively. Perhaps most importantly, they didn't consume it alone, they didn't consume the alcohol *to consume alcohol*, it was consumed with a higher intention, a higher intention of connecting more deeply with their community.

All these caveats ran through my head as I bounced along the dance floor, swept up in the infectious smiles of the locals around me who sweated and sung with the music. It was truly the "best party I've ever been to."

Perhaps it wasn't about the wine at all.

But, then again, without the wine I wonder if it would be the same…

Movement

"Movement is life."

*-Paul Chek, Renowned trainer
& spiritual teacher*

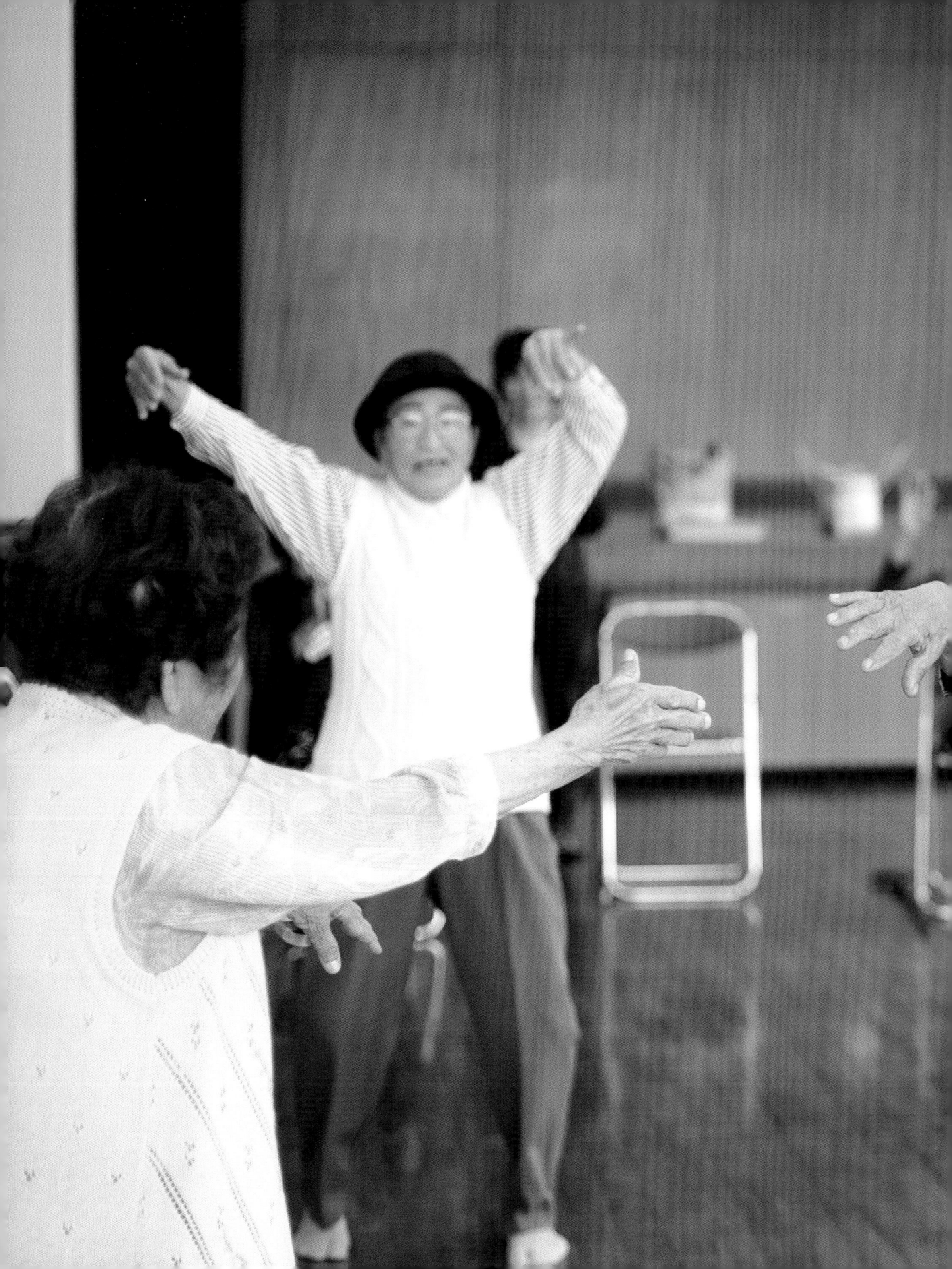

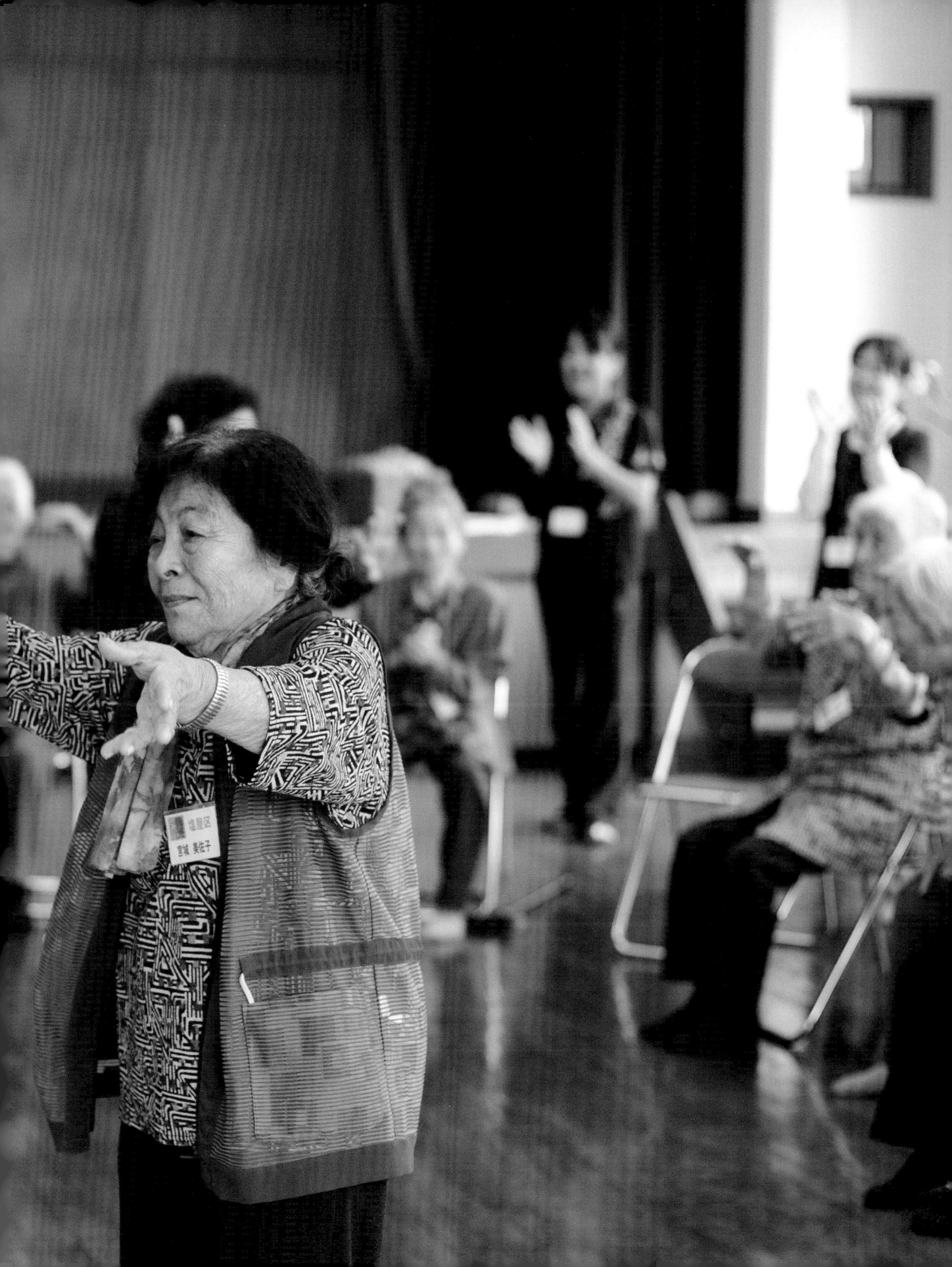

Australians sit down for an average of ten hours per day. After about four hours of sitting in one day, our capacity for burning fat and clearing the body of toxins is diminished.

Physical stagnation is not something that the longevity cultures experience. There is a strong theme of constant physical activity in these regions, be it harvesting food from one's garden or taking a nature walk with friends and family.

As Paul Chek explained to me in California, physical movement pumps lymphatic fluid around the body, strengthens muscles, increases bone density and overall this leads to a healthier existence. Hip fractures are one of the top killers of people over the age of sixty-five and most of these could be prevented by simple movement practices applied in one's life every single day.

You've heard a lot of this before, I know *but*, movement in the longevity cultures? It's different.

When you mention *movement*, most people think of their exercise routine; the gym, yoga, pilates or going for a run. In the longevity cultures *movement* is equated with *life*. In Ikaria, one can expect to climb dozens of steep stairs throughout the day in order to achieve daily tasks. Added to which are the people's gardening chores, social and work obligations which all incite movement.

In Okinawa, people's social schedules demand that they spend a large portion of the day moving between locations on foot, climbing stairs, dancing and singing (not to mention the gardening!).

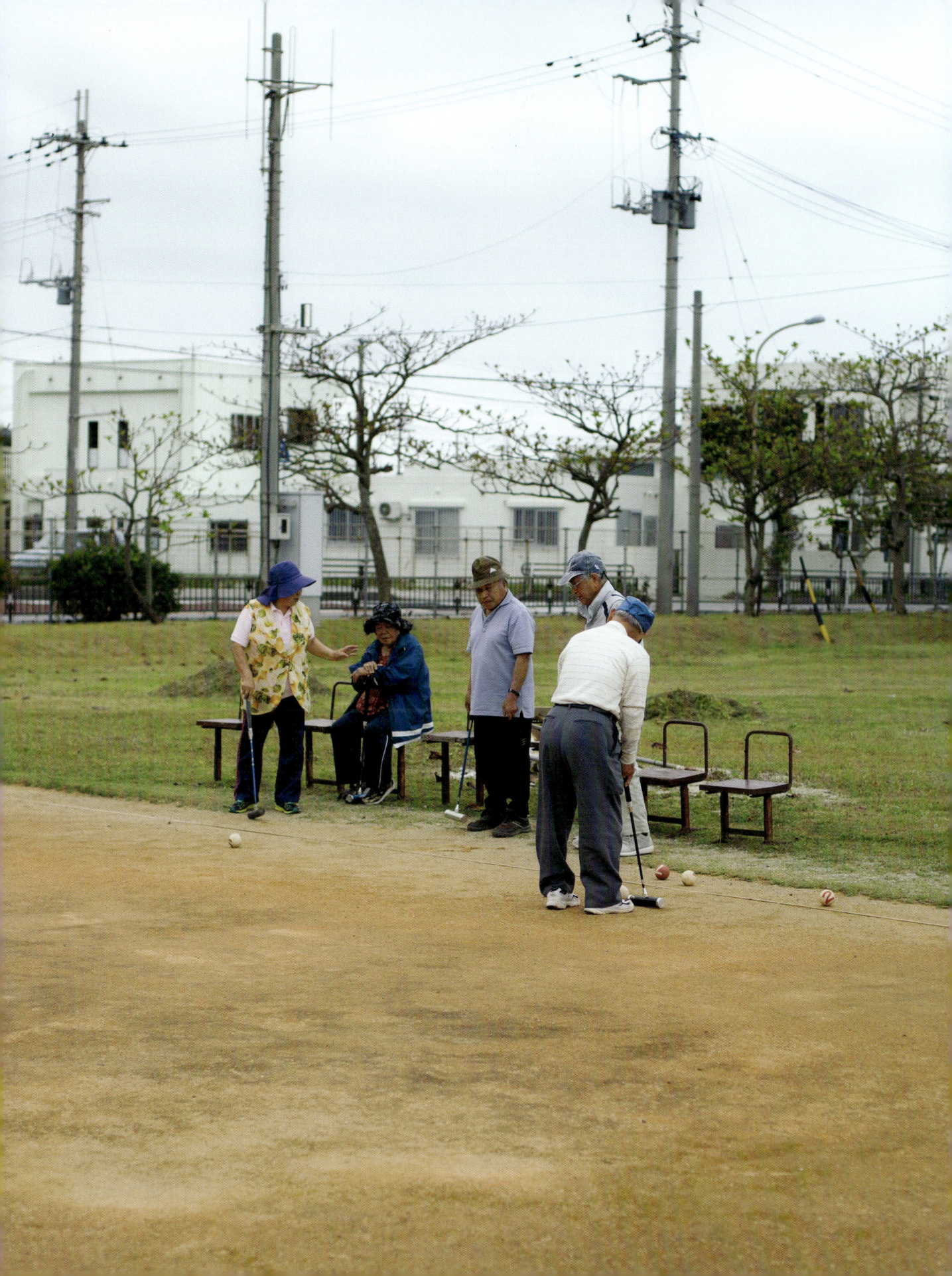

"There's a saying in Okinawa that the children and parents should live close enough so that the younger generation can make soup at home and then walk it over to the parents' house without it getting cold. So, close, but not too close."

-Dr. Craig Wilcox, medical anthropologist

As part of the Seventh-day Adventist religion, a weekly sabbath is implemented into people's lives in Loma Linda. This means that from Friday sundown until Saturday sundown time is taken to relax, connect with friends and family, and to prepare for a Sunday service. Often, this time is spent on a nature walk which is encouraged in their scriptures.

The key idea here is that movement is *embedded* into the longevity cultures' way of life. In 'the West', we have to carve time out of our lives to move, whereas in the blue zones it is simply a part of every day living.

People in these regions aren't smashing themselves at the gym for a half hour in the morning and then going to work to sit for the rest of the day. They are burning the candle slowly, naturally, squatting to pick some weeds, lunging as they climb steep stairs, twisting and bending as they dance or pick up children, pulling and pushing as they fix something on the farm or in the house - they *move naturally every single day* and avoid spending too much time sitting.

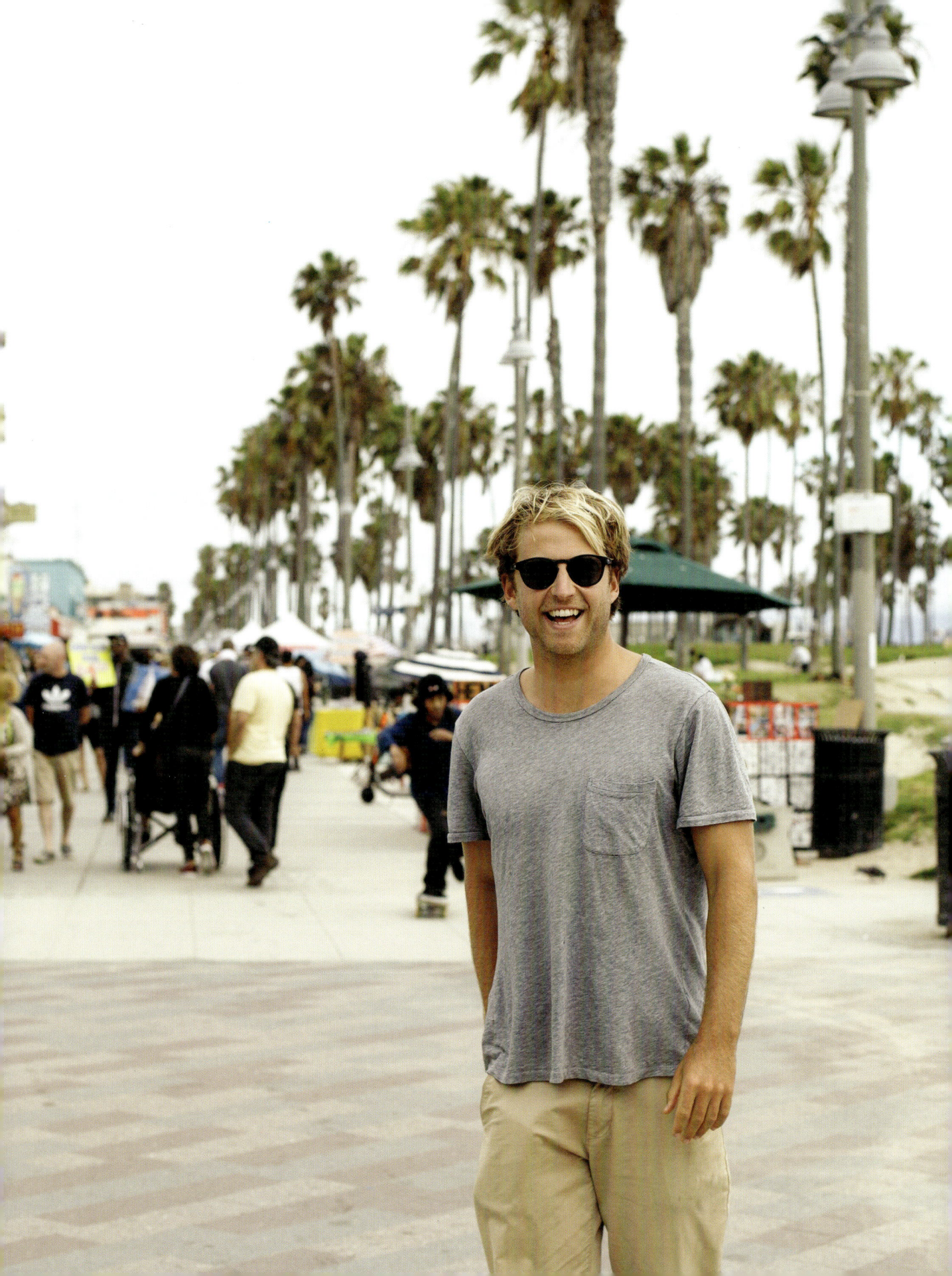

We can implement this pillar into our own lives using a few simple techniques.

Shopping
The next time you go shopping, either walk to the store with your grocery bags or park as far away as possible to induce some walking.

Get a dog... or a mate!
We are far more likely to spend time moving if we have a degree of accountability. Having a pet who needs a walk or a friend who will join you are great strategies to implement more natural movement into your life.

At work
Have several different 'working' positions that you can move into throughout the day as opposed to staying in one chair for eight hours. I like to use a Swiss ball for this where I can sit on top with my knees folded underneath, I can sit cross legged or just bounce lightly in a normal seated position whilst working. Furthermore, if you have phone calls or meetings to conduct, ask those involved if you might do them whilst walking outside in the sunshine - walking meetings are an addiction, trust me!

Your location

When I arrived home from my trip overseas, I knew I needed to move house. The location we were in was too isolated from the daily essentials which were, for me, the surf, a good cafe and friends (all in one!). We ended up shifting one suburb over and now have everything within walking distance, from the local beekeeper to the organic store and some pumping surf! I went to fill up my car with petrol the other day and it had spider webs over the petrol cap!

We age to the degree that we allow ourselves to become immobile or dysfunctional. As Dr. Mark Hyman said in my interview with him, *muscle loss is the disease of ageing.* By staying limber, active, strong and agile we ensure the quality and quantity of our years on this earth.

Community

"You have 50% less risk of dying early if you have strong links to family and friends. On the flip side, social isolation and withdrawal are worse for us than smoking, obesity and substance abuse. We're just discovering the power of strong social & familial connection. It turns out 'that feeling' of being accepted by our tribe is the key to a long, happy & healthy life."

-Dr. Ali Walker, social scientist

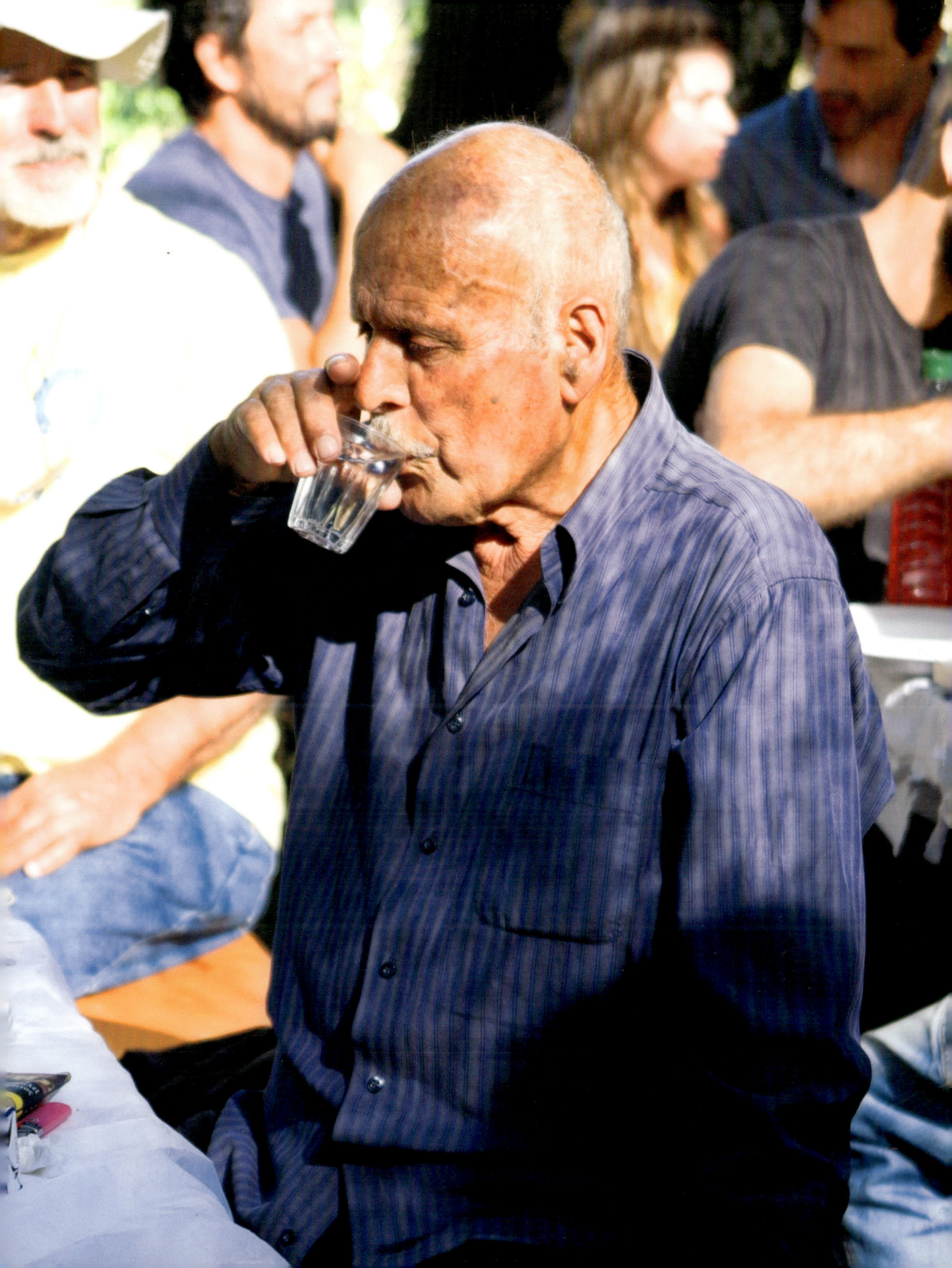

Ikaria; The Panagiri

On one of our last night's in Ikaria we were invited to a _panagiri_, a local religious festival. We arrived at 10am, we didn't leave until 11pm. The panagiri is set up within each community and takes place at a local square or church. In the beginning, religious services are held followed by truckloads, literally, of food and wine. We watched as about 1000L of home-made, organic and definitely preservative free red wine was delivered on the back of a tiny lorry. It backed up into the square with the wine separated into 1L plastic bottles and piled into open crates which we then carried into the hall.

Right by the hall, a massive steel drum, the biggest crockpot I've ever seen, holds about 700kg of wild goat all slow cooking in water. The warm, fatty broth is spooned out and served to anybody who wants it, the tender meat is taken inside to be sold to all the attendees of the festival alongside locally grown organic produce. Beautifully, the profit generated from the _panagiri_ is then distributed within the village as the community sees fit, a dilapidated road, a school classroom, a particular family doing it tough, the insular island economics are certainly socially-driven.

This economic set up really defines the community-mindedness of the longevity cultures. In Okinawa, a Moai social group is established at a very young age and might last 90+ years. Money is brought to Moai meetings and distributed on a needs basis. In Loma Linda, a seventh day adventist congregation is _all about community_, be it feeding the homeless, talking about God or simply being there to ask someone "how are you?".

It was one of the most beautiful travel experiences I've ever had, the *panagiri*, because I got to truly delve into the local culture as a welcomed guest, not a tourist. The deep sense of present state awareness brought to the event was as tangible as the loud Greek music played by the local band to the dozens of people on the dance floor. People talked to each other, smiled, mingled with those 80 years younger or older and often came up to me, completely without a lick of English, just to smile and shake my hand before walking by.

Beekeeper George was there and he danced the night away, as nimble as any nightclub goer I'd seen back home. George and I swapped partners several times but in the end he got annoyed at me for "stealing all of the women", as he put it, and sat back down to drink wine and eat salad with his friends.

As the dance floor became more and more densely populated, I sat back down to simply observe what was going on in front of me. No phones, music just loud enough to lose yourself in the dance but still chat with the person opposite, organic local food and wine, grandchildren, grandparents, parents, sisters, brothers, husbands and wives, all intermingled and deep in conversation or laughter while the glorious sun offered a bedazzling light display, penetrating the leafy trees surrounding the church square.

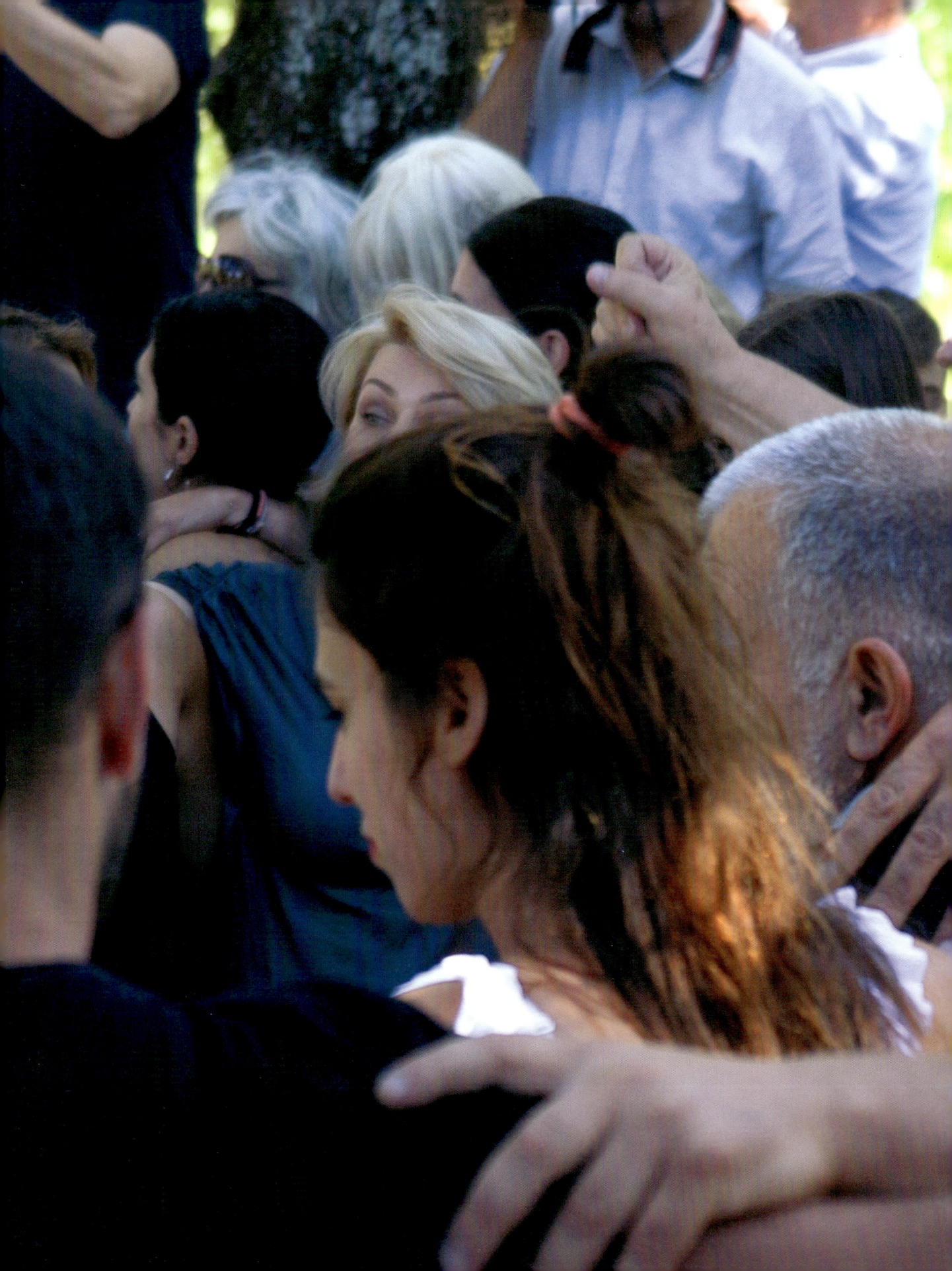

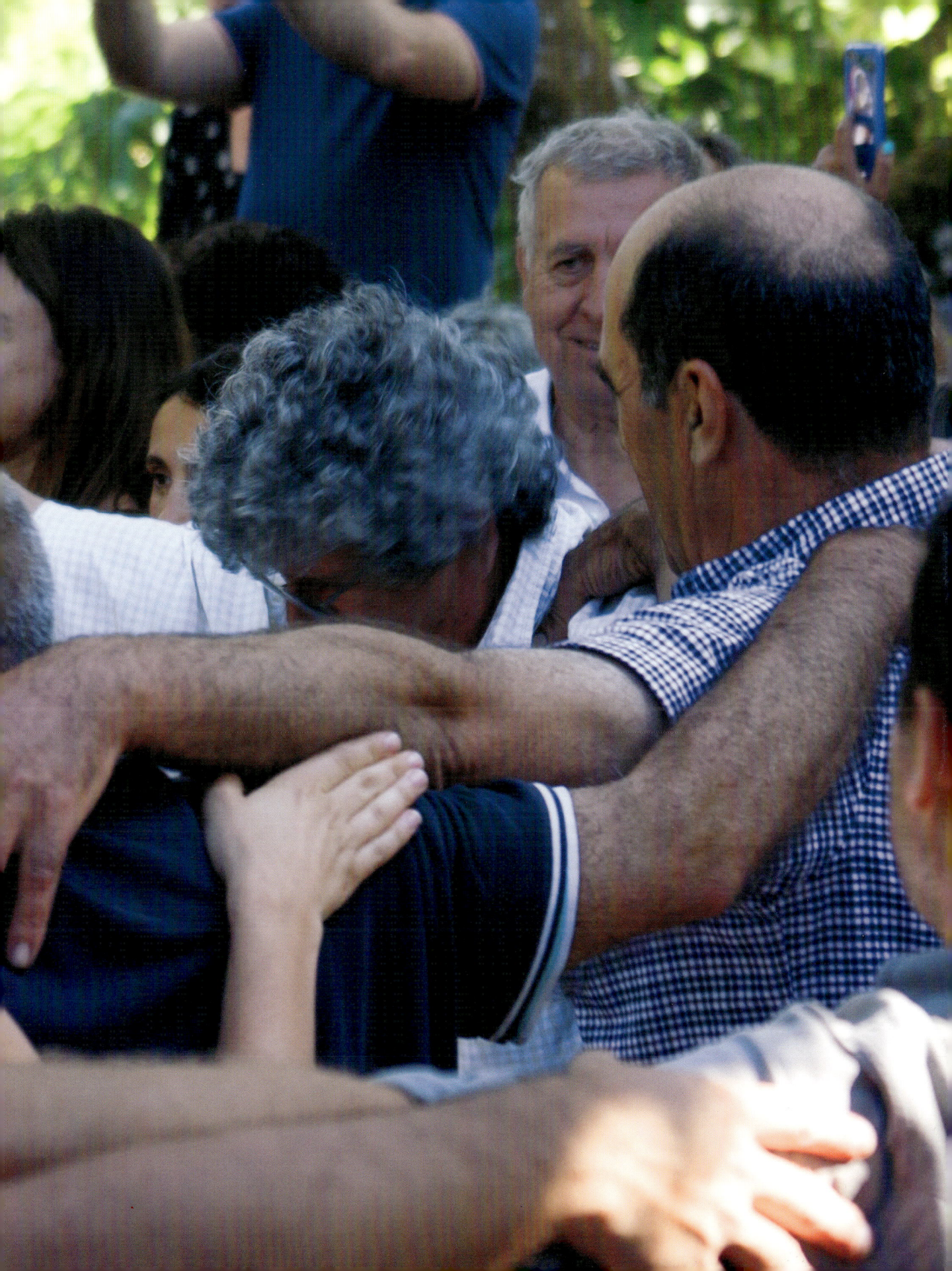

Coupled with my warm sense of awe was a calm, gentle feeling of sadness. This sort of thing didn't happen back home, or in many other places around the world. We have fallen for the allure of the short, fast, instant gratification regarding food, socialising, technology, money & more. We no longer appreciate the slow, calm, stoic, persistent approach to life, like that which was being displayed in front of me at the panagiri.

Many people in western societies think their community exists in their smartphone and by scrolling through their social media feeds somehow they 'check' the very important box of *community*. This is not the case.

"Studies show that we don't get the same benefits from a text that we do from talking with someone on the phone or seeing them face to face."

-Dr. Ali Walker, social scientist

"Just a couple thousand years ago, which is not that long, we lived in hunter gatherer clans made up of related or interdependent individuals. That, from a community perspective, worked very well. Now, with our modern technology, we've been broken down from communities, to families and now to an individual level.

We don't know our neighbours anymore. There's no sense of shared fate anymore, so there's less incentive to look after one another.

If community is the most important piece, then we really need to put some focus there."

-Daniel Vitalis, writer & speaker

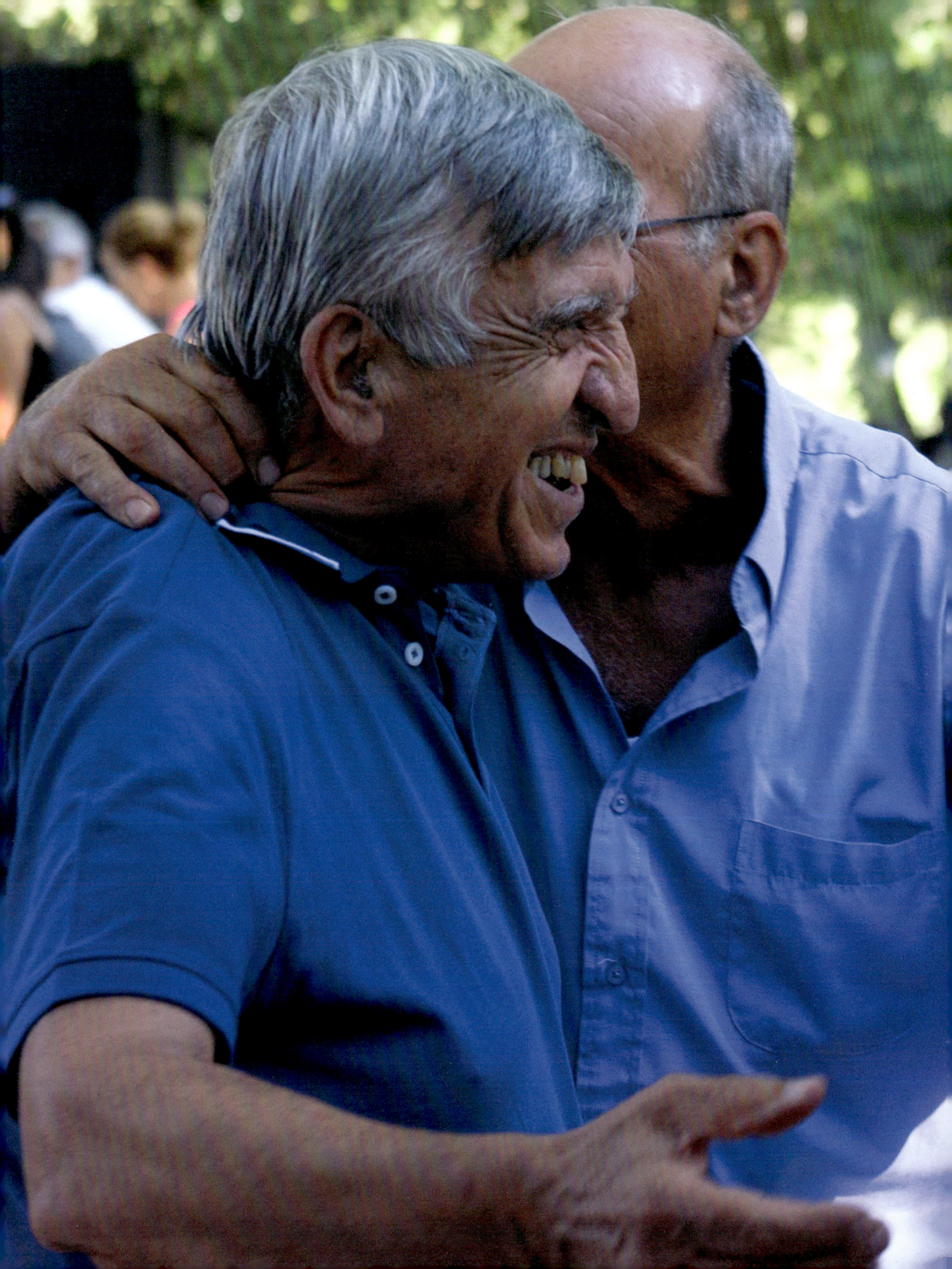

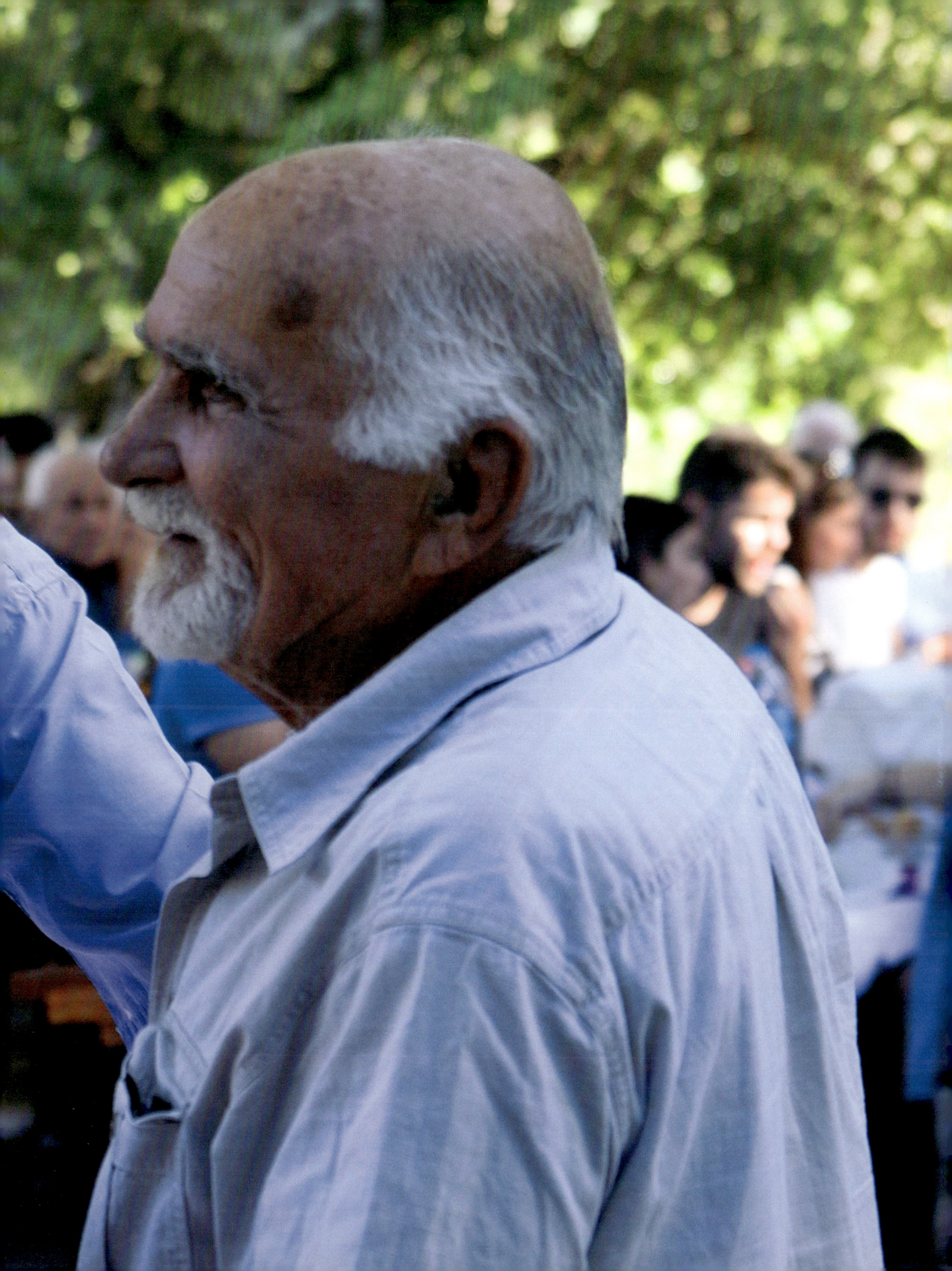

In the blue zones, people have a very strong sense of community. When I spoke with Thea in Ikaria, she said that because the population on the island is so small, everybody knows each other. The result of this situation is that there is a sense of accountability with one's actions because 'if you do something bad everyone will know about it.'

We need to re-approximate our own versions of these communities in our own lives. I say re-approximate instead of 'mimic' because it is impossible for most of us to live in a society where everybody knows each other; our cities are simply too big for that. What we can do, though, is create sub-communities amongst our towns, our suburbs, even our streets or apartment buildings. By developing a shared sense of fate, of ownership and accountability of a geographical area we can break down the inherent awkwardness of getting to know strangers. These relationships often progress from 'acquaintance' to 'friends' quite quickly and can offer a very tangible buffer for the human need to socialise and feel safe in a community.

In my home town on the northern beaches of Sydney, I surround myself with friends of all ages. We are mostly likeminded (this isn't essential), we participate in the same activities such as surfing and the creative arts, but more importantly we've created a situation where we bump into each other constantly. On the street, in the surf, in a cafe or on the yoga mat! This is important because, in today's busy times, trying to 'force' a scheduled 'community appointment' can sometimes feel a little inauthentic and awkward. By creating a lifestyle where you 'can't walk down the street without bumping into someone' we can actually enjoy a beautiful situation that is set up for a feeling of safety, security and engagement with our community!

To better appreciate the third essential pillar of longevity and wellness, you can do a few things.

Develop daily habits

So you enjoy going out for a coffee every day? Frequent the same one or two cafes when you do it. Naturally, you'll begin to connect with the staff at the cafe who will ask you about your day, they'll comment on the weather, the sports and other current events which will eventually lead to deeper and more meaningful connection. You'll also begin to recognise and chat with regular customers, one of whom might just be your next best friend!

Join a social group

You can skip a few steps on the friendship progression scale by simply joining some sort of social group. Perhaps it's a volunteering group, such as the one I worked with in Loma Linda who fed the homeless once per week, perhaps it's a walking group or a swimming group. These organised time commitments create a sense of accountability and group connection quickly and can obliterate the typical gauntlets you must cross when meeting new people.

Use social media wisely

I find that many people outside of longevity cultures feel 'too tired and worn out' to socialise. I believe this is because we not only spend too much time working, but also because we engage with social media too often. By creating a 'knowledge buffer' between you and your community, you can trick yourself into feeling more curious about what people are up to in their life, thus energising you to stay social. By limiting time on social media, we also avoid that 'drained, let down' feeling that is typical of any social media use.

Stay present

Whilst connecting with friends, family or your community, ensure that you stay *in the moment*. When you ask someone how their day is going, *listen* to their answer. Engaging someone in meaningful conversation means that you speak *and* listen. When you participate in meaningful conversation there is a deluge of positive neurochemicals which flood your system and deliver outstanding health benefits.

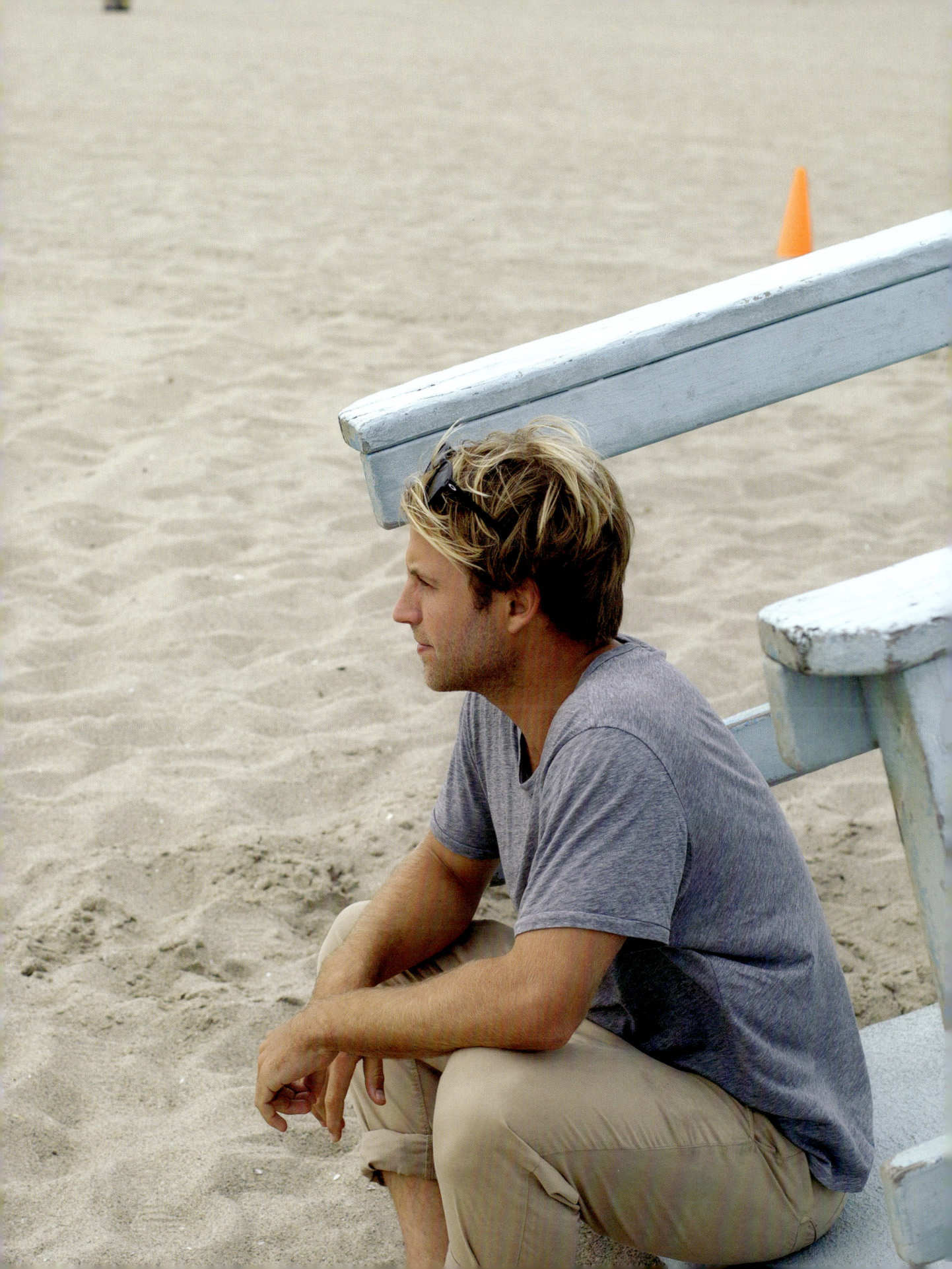

Attitude

Of the four pillars of longevity & wellness, what I found most tangible during my time with the graceful agers was their *attitude.*

Okinawa, Japan

At 97 years old, Chosei Hentona is cheeky. We arrived at his humble, garden-rich abode to find him sitting lazily in the sun, basking in his work overalls with a small bucket hat atop his head. He jumped up and grinned sharply as we approached.

Saori, my Japanese producer, introduced me and he sized me up comically.

"America?"

"No," Saori corrected. "Australia."

"I am going to sit."

"Okay, can we take some pictures?"

"Sure, I may smoke a cigarette. I'm not sure yet."

"What sort of cigarettes do you smoke?"

"I can't remember, the smoky ones."

I laughed and he guffawed animatedly.

"How many cigarettes do you have each day?"

"I don't know, I started in WW2 because everybody else did it and kept asking why I didn't. It stuck. All I know is in the morning I smoke and then go to the toilet. It's my routine."

Fair enough. We watched on, taking some photographs and capturing footage as Chosei squatted deeply in his garden, manually tilling the soil before he planted some new seedlings. The soil looked rich as it sifted into the light and fell back down with each flick of Chosei's spade.

He worked at this, seemingly indefatigable for ten minutes before mumbling something about being finished and then made his way back over to us. There was a deep presence about him. He was completely unrushed and undeterred by our big production camera and smiling, fascinated faces.

"You look strong," he observed objectively, looking me up and down and laughing at my reaction when Saori translates. He called animatedly to Saori once again, he wanted to challenge me to a pushup competition on the paved garden path.

Laughing at each other whilst doing so, we proceeded to complete 5 pushups in unison before he (gratefully on my part) stopped. Totally unaffected and with no noticeable change in breath, he told me he did one armed push ups until he was 90 and then had to stop.

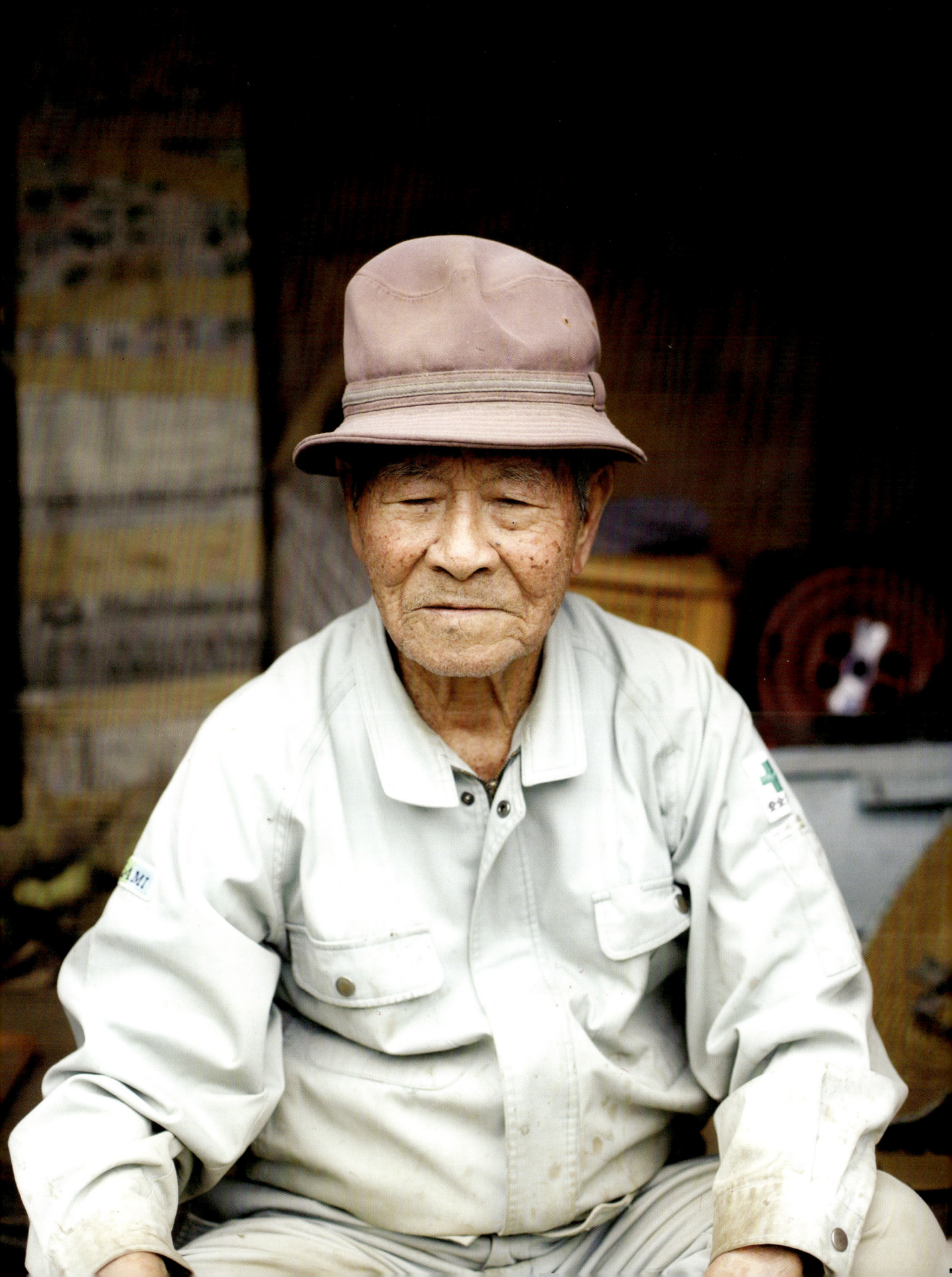

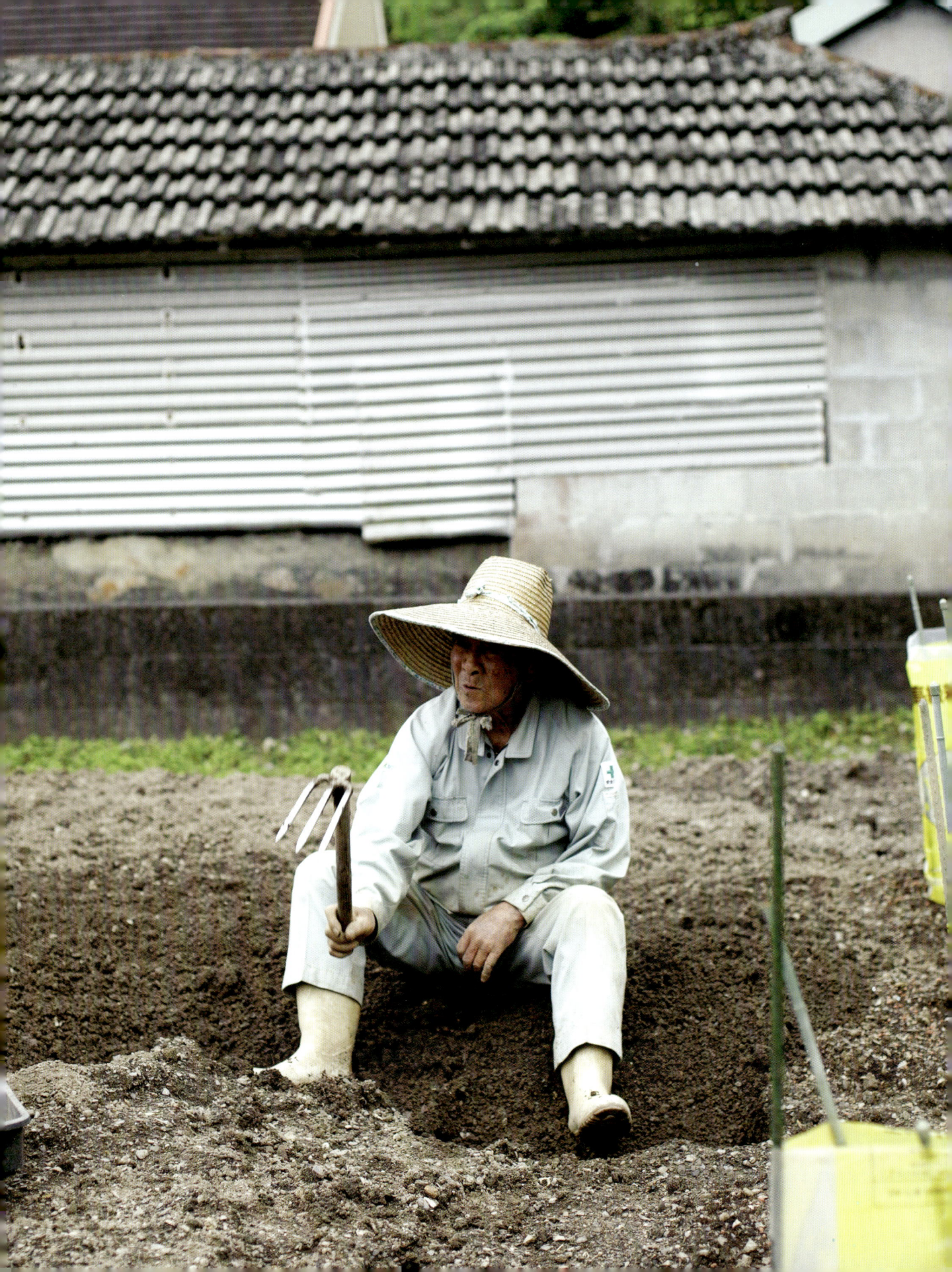

"That's incredible," I replied. "How are you still so healthy at 97? Is there a secret?"

Chosei smacks his lips a few times in deep thought before arriving at a prophetic answer.

"Not sure. I just never died."

All of the people that I met in the longevity cultures had a great attitude toward life. They were stoic in a way, smug even, and brought such an overarching sense of confidence that it made me just want to be around them.

As we know from recent scientific research, the mind and body are intimately connected. In fact, this phenomena has been discussed throughout history all the way back to Hippocrates' time, but the recent evidence suggests that the way we *think* and approach life determines to a large extent our physical expression of health.

Many of the blue zone inhabitants have a challenging history which they have lived through. In Okinawa, the island was ravaged for many years during World War Two. It was bombed with thousands of people dying as a result. Many of the people I met there lived through the experience and could recall it clearly.

War has also impacted Ikaria over time. I spoke with a local beekeeper, Yorigo (George), who recalled how many people on the island died from starvation due to import restrictions during the war. If people weren't growing their own produce, and enough of it, they died.

It would be easy to note these experiences and expect to find a traumatised, begrudging people in existence today, but it's the complete opposite. The people in these longevity cultures are happy, delightfully so, and look back on such times as momentous teachers of humility, faith and perseverance. It also reminds them to be grateful for peaceful modern times and to be deeply present in each day, without overthinking the past or future.

People in longevity cultures live a purposeful life. They know why they get up in the morning. In Okinawa this is known as one's *ikigai*, a reason for living, and all of the graceful agers whom I interviewed could clearly articulate their ikigai as soon as I asked them to. Many talked about family and friends, many talked about having 'too many things to do' and some just talked about having fun and being happy. If you have a higher purpose for which you exist, it will add years to your life.

Having a clear purpose leads to an attitude of strong will, it leads to a clarity of priorities in life and develops a significant amount of emotional resilience. When people are resilient, they are more humble, affable and contented, and this was certainly the case with the people I met in Okinawa, Ikaria & Loma Linda.

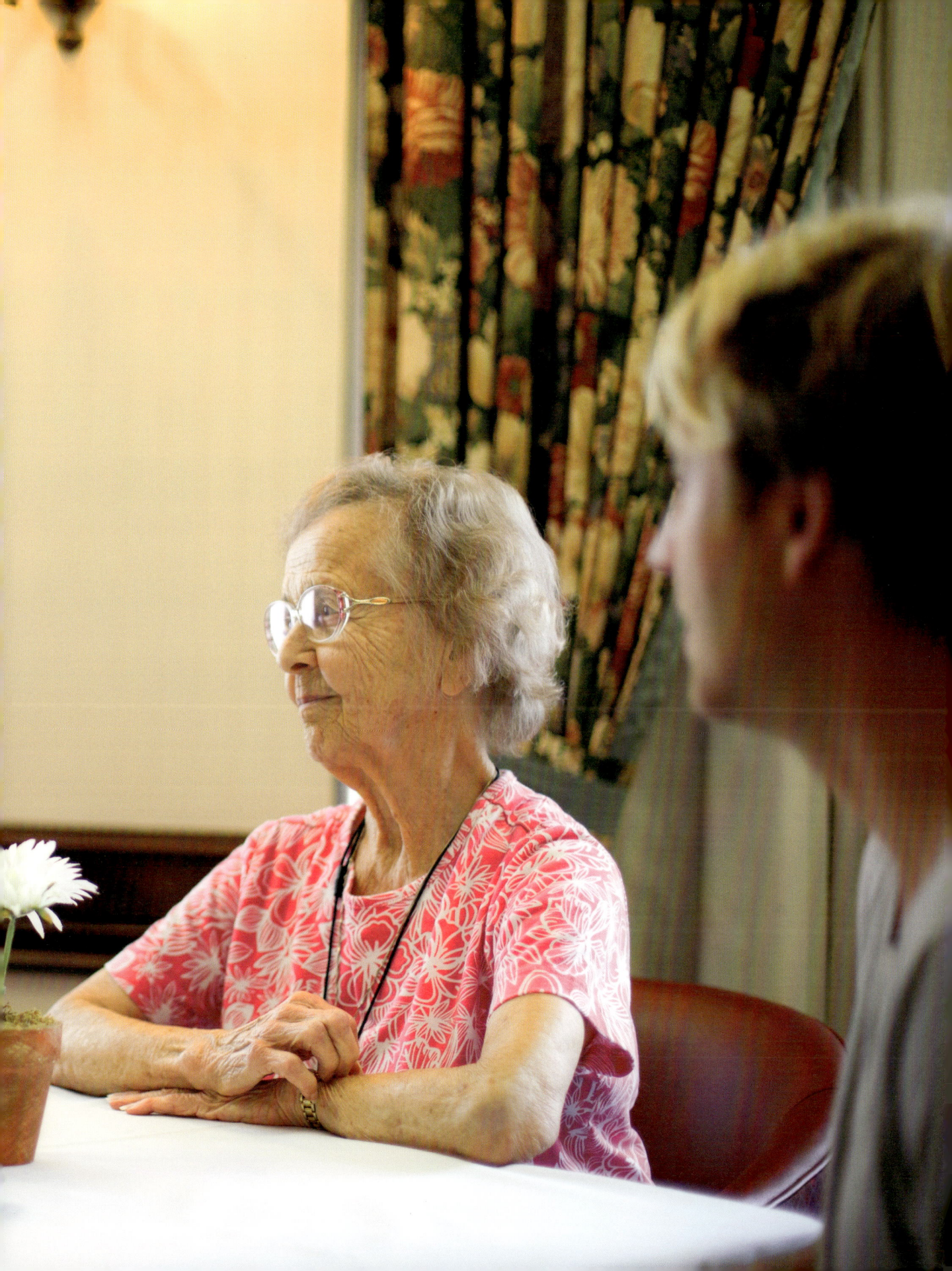

Loma Linda, California

My throat constricted in agony, my eyes watered, my muscles ached and my head pounded in the harsh sunshine glaring down upon the Loma Linda University campus. I was sick.

What had started as a slight tickle in my throat at the beginning of a plane ride some twenty hours ago had turned into one of the worst flus I had ever experienced. I had spent the night shivering uncontrollably, sipping at my water bottle and questioning my career choice miserably in our hotel room down by the beach. Now, I had come to see one of the world's healthiest suburbs, as if to throw it in my face that my new age yoga and green smoothies approach to wellness was still falling short of the longevity culture experience.

I wanted to go home. I didn't want to be here. _Why can't someone else do this crap?_ I whined.

We conducted interviews on campus and were taught the fundamentals of the Loma Lindan way of life. Vegetarianism, a weekly sabbath, an integrative medical school, yep - I get it, _now take me home_ I glumly thought.

That afternoon I was taken to a local church. I met Mike, one of the happiest people in the world, who is a pastor at the church and is in his thirties. He sipped cooly at a steaming coffee as we arrived and was dressed in a stylish button up, blue denims and skate shoes.

"Welcome man!"

His energetic and bubbly attitude forced me to try and match him at his level, despite my physiological woes.

"What are we going to do today?" I asked, chasing down a true, authentic Loma Lindan experience. "Can you take me on a nature walk? Can we do a pot luck?"

"We're actually going to be doing some community outreach work tonight man. We're putting on some food and drink for the homeless people in the area."

Before we knew it, we were ushered into a room out the back of the church. A growing line of people waited outside to enter, these people, Mike explained, had fallen on tough times and were currently homeless in the area. Some had been for decades.

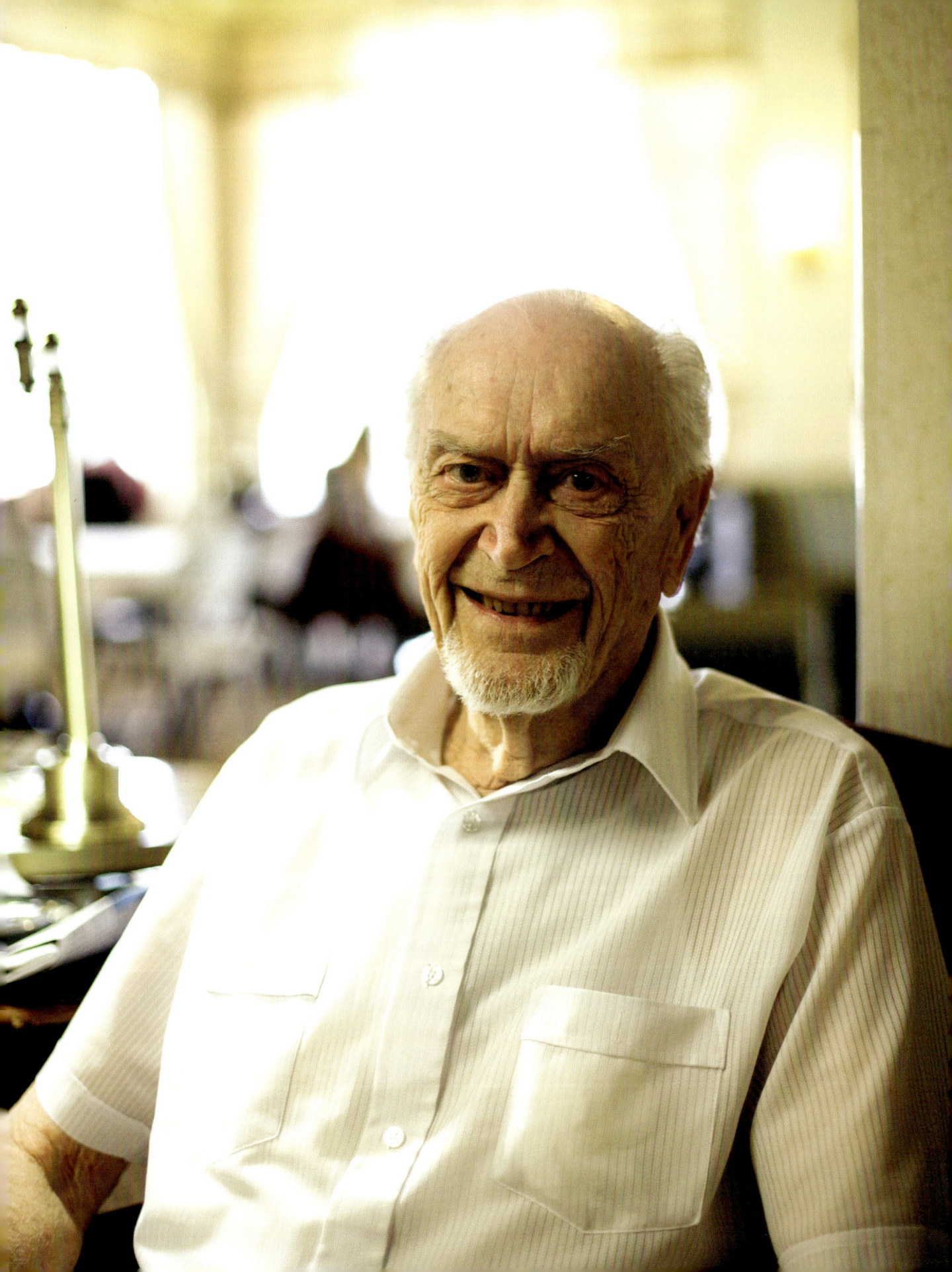

We stood in a circle before getting to work, a group meeting of sorts where some prayers were offered. Then, I was put to work serving lasagne and salad to the seemingly endless string of people waiting, one hand outstretched balancing a paper plate and some cutlery, for a meal.

Gradually, I started to feel better. I began conversing with the people in the room. I told them about Australia, they told me about America. And suddenly I couldn't even remember that I was supposed to be sick. My throat ache began diminishing and my aching head calmed down to the point that twenty minutes later I felt like a new person. I'd never, ever, had such a miraculous turn around in my health in such a short amount of time.

That was when I realised the power of a good attitude. The power of giving, the power that comes from directly helping others less fortunate than yourself. In the longevity cultures, these opportunities to help others in some way, to lend a hand (*mostly non financial*) to someone who needs it are frequent and fruitful.

"If someone is brave enough to ask for help it creates an opportunity for someone else to be good. Without them, the opportunity doesn't exist.

I daresay that proper purpose has the capacity to change not just your life, but the lives of those around you. If everybody knew what their purpose was, we would all connect in such an unbridled, beautiful way.

Science has shown there are so many physiological and psychological benefits to helping people. Living longer, less heart disease, less stress and a huge release of positive feel good chemicals in the body."

-Seb Terry, author & speaker

I had allowed my circumstance to dictate my emotions in those first hours in Loma Linda. I had created a feedback loop which had reinforced those negative feelings each time my inner dialogue justified my emotions. It took me *helping someone else* to break that loop.

We're told that we can fix our attitude with medicines these days but I truly believe that medicines will never 'cure' us from our mental health challenges. We can never replace the healing power of engaging with other people, of living with purpose, of moving naturally every day, of eating a seasonal, local and organic diet with a pill.

You can develop a resilient, humble and affable attitude by applying these tools into your life.

The right people
Surround yourself with people who encourage you to be yourself. Community is fantastic, when you have the right one! If you feel like you can't express yourself openly within yours, then you need to find a new one. In the longevity cultures, people spend their time with each other laughing, telling stories, sharing their controversial opinions on various topics and lightly teasing each other. These playful experiences with others will help you develop a strong, resilient attitude to bring with you into life.

Help someone else

Volunteering in some way has been shown to be an incredible emotional health tool. By exposing yourself to the sometimes harsh realities of the world, you can gain new perspectives on your own situation and potentially even garner an attitude of gratitude. If you don't have time to volunteer, try to go above and beyond in your working life and see how that service impacts the lives of your clients or fellow employees.

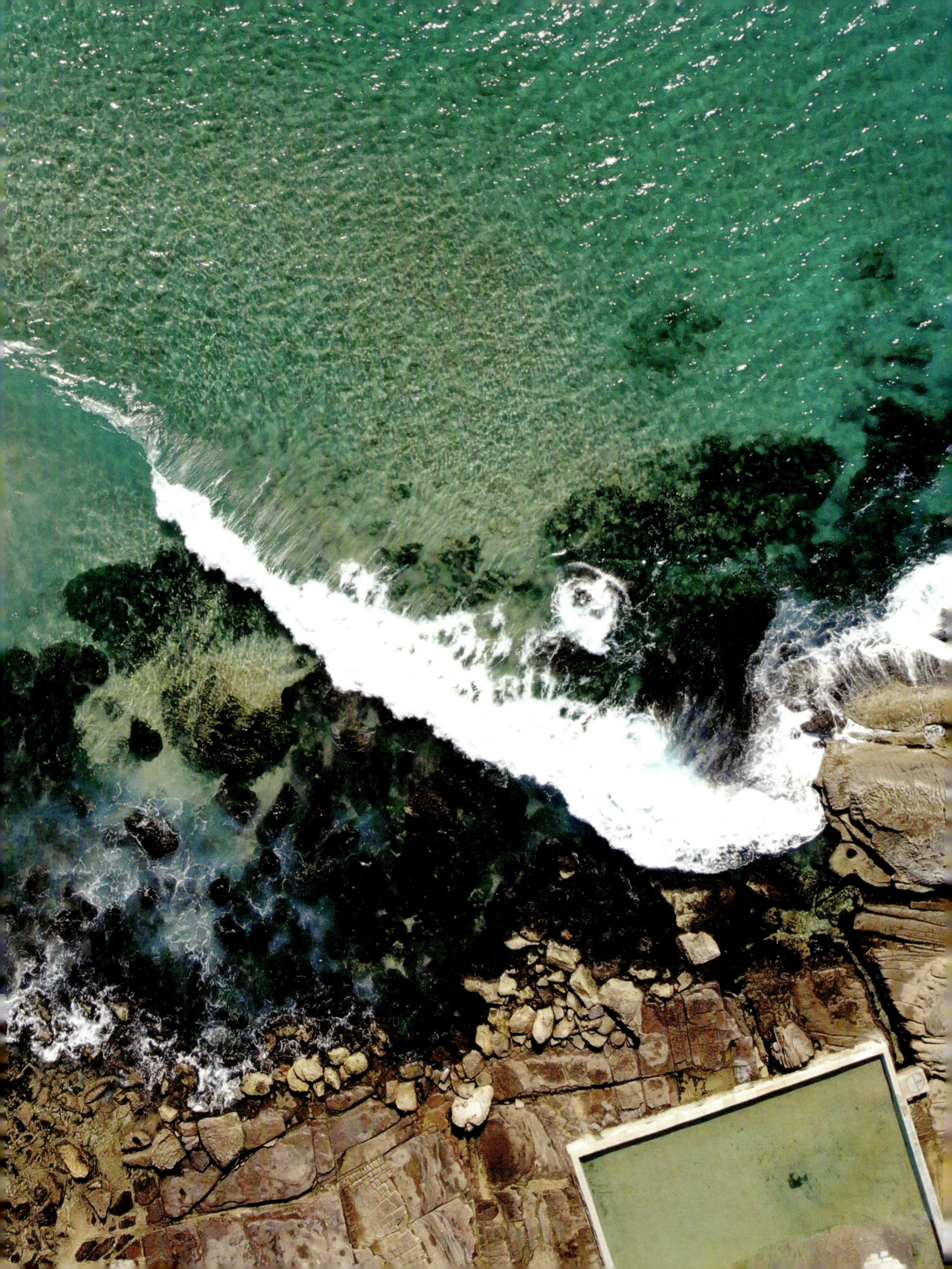

Sydney, Australia

The plane touches down, smoothly and safely without a wobble, and I'm thankful to be back in Sydney, Australia, my home town. I nervously brush the laptop section of my backpack, inside which resides about $100k's worth of footage and photos documenting the last month on the road. It's all there, safe and sound. My production camera is above me in the overhead locker and I frown as I haul it out, the heavy, black, awkward case a poetic reflection of the equipment's place in my life and business at the moment. I will sell it, I have decided, alongside all of my other professional production equipment. I will no longer self fund production projects; this is my first determined step toward adopting a longevity lifestyle.

Weathered, red-eyed and quiet, I gaze out into the miserable rainy weather in Sydney as the airport shuttle inches painstakingly along the M5, hauling myself and my $100k hard drive up to the Northern Beaches. I hear beeping, I see stressed out drivers on their way to work in a job that, statistically, they probably hate in order to pay for a home that's bigger and fancier than they probably need. I see people sacrificing their health, their relationships, their _time_ for a false promise we've been made that if we earn a little more, have a little more, we'll be better off. We won't.

I'm saddened by the knowledge that, one month ago, I left behind what are probably the most important and healthy things in life, just to go and find out what the most important and healthy things are.

It's my partner, my family and my community. It's my local environment, my somewhat pathetic attempt at a garden on my small apartment balcony, it's the people who serve me at my local health cafe, the friends who I see in the water surfing.

These realisations cause me to wonder if I should quit, leave it all behind, the dreams, the starry lights of film making and the glory of story telling. Right now, feeling deeply exhausted both physically and emotionally, it seems like an attractive idea, but then Beekeeper George's advice runs through my head.

"Everything in moderation. You can't enjoy rest if you're not tired."

-George, beekeeper in Ikaria

About the author

Kale Brock is a writer and filmmaker. He lives in Sydney and spends his time surfing, working, spending time with friends and traveling.

His documentaries, The Gut Movie and The Longevity Film, have generated international acclaim whilst his books, The Gut Healing Protocol, The Art Of Probiotic Nutrition & Mandy Microbe's Big Gut Adventure have gone on to become international bestsellers.

You can join Kale on social media @kalesbroccoli

You can watch Kale's films and purchase books at kalebrock.com

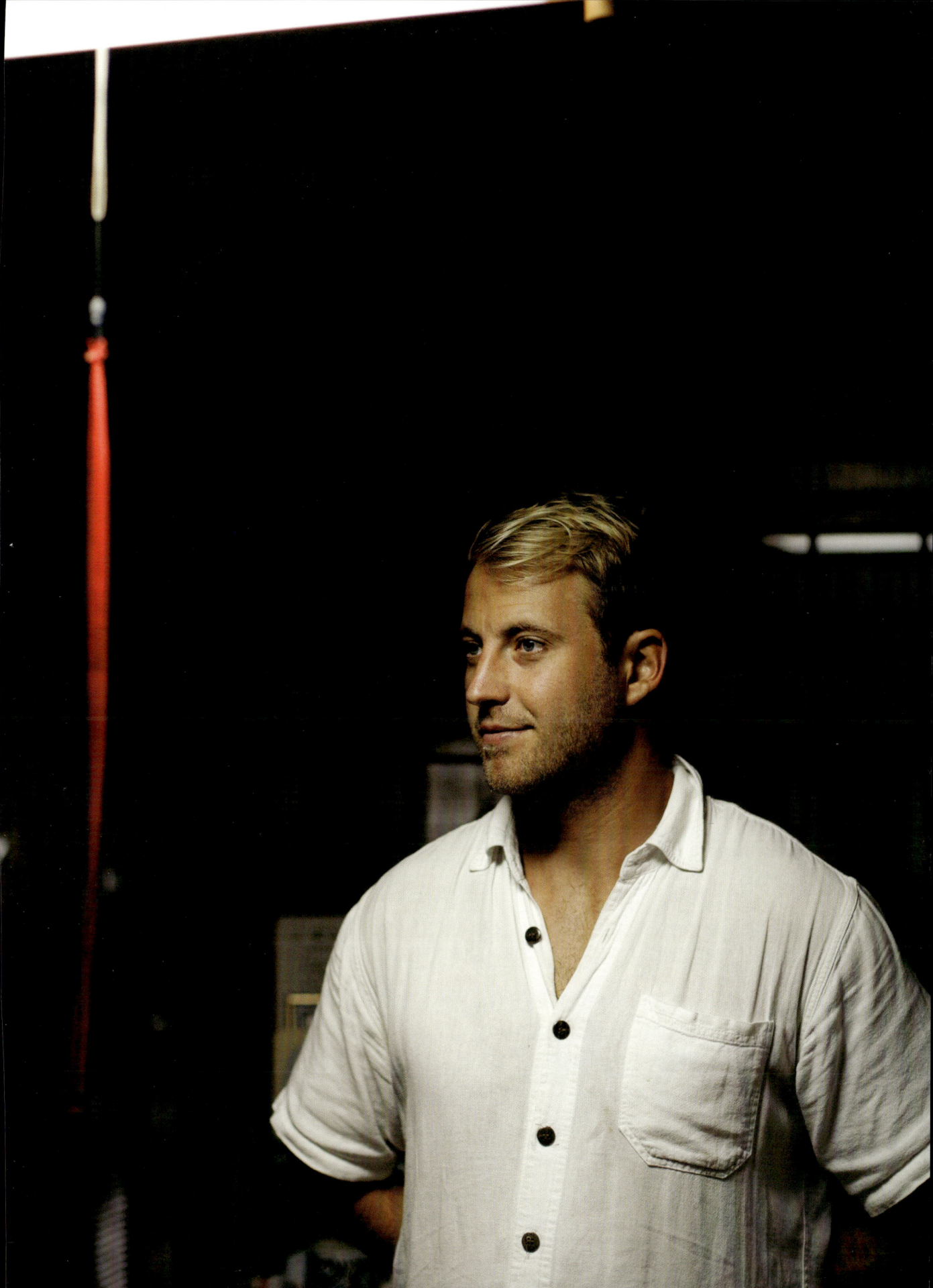